THE KAJI REVIEW

Emergency Medicine Clinical Review Book

Volume 3

Amy H. Kaji MD PhD

Professor of Clinical Medicine
Harbor-UCLA Medical Center
Department of Emergency Medicine

Associate Editors

Jaskaran Singh MD
Harbor-UCLA Medical Center
Department of Emergency Medicine

Daniel G. Ostermayer MD
Assistant Professor of Emergency Medicine
University of Texas Health Science Center at Houston
McGovern Medical School

Assistant Editors

Amit Suneja MD MPH
Harbor-UCLA Medical Center
Department of Emergency Medicine

Lauren Fryling, MD
Harbor-UCLA Medical Center
Department of Emergency Medicine

Ronald Luu MD
Harbor-UCLA Medical Center
Department of Emergency Medicine

Null Publishing
Group

Null Publishing Group, an independent academic publisher, provides tools, resources, and expertise to authors publishing educational texts. Authors retain ownership, control, and copyright of their published works and gain the flexibility and power of digital publishing. For more information visit http://nullpublishing.com or email info@nullpublishing.com.

Types of non-arrhythmogenic syncope		
Mechanical	Vasovagal (reflex, neurally mediated, or neurocardiogenic)	Orthostatic (postural)

Causes include:
• Valvular dysfunction
 	
• Myocardial dysfunction
 	
• Severe heart failure
 	
• Hypertrophic cardiomyopathy
 	
• Pericardial disease (tamponade)
 	
• Vascular etiologies:
  • Pulmonary embolism
  • Aortic dissection
	This results in a **cardioinhibitory response leading to bradycardia and a vasodepressor response leading to hypotension.**
	
	Common triggers include:
	• Phlebotomy
	• Micturition
	• Defication
		Hypotension associated with:
		• Change in body position
		
		• Dehydration
		
		• Autonomic insufficiency (e.g. Parkinson's disease, diabetes mellitus)
		
		• Alcohol use
		
		• Medications (e.g. antihypertensives, opiates, psychoactive drugs)

• Weiner RB et al. Case 25-2018: A 63 year old man with syncope. NEJM 2018;379:670-80.

Null Publishing Group

Null Publishing Group, an independent academic publisher, provides tools, resources, and expertise to authors publishing educational texts. Authors retain ownership, control, and copyright of their published works and gain the flexibility and power of digital publishing. For more information visit http://nullpublishing.com or email info@nullpublishing.com.

The Kaji Review

Welcome to the Kaji Review. This book is intended for students, residents, advanced practitioners, and senior physicians alike. Although formatted as a question book, the Kaji Review is really an evidence-based clinical case book to advance your bedside knowledge and clinical expertise.

Content pulls heavily from textbooks and LLSA readings. Topics are focused on emergency care but also cover outpatient and inpatient medical and surgical topics. Often the explanations include textbook references, evidence-based guidelines, online resources, and specific details of clinical research. The references are intended to be used as a reading list for high quality primary literature.

Please enjoy Volumes 1 and 2 as well.

- Volume 1
- Volume 2

CARDIOLOGY

#1

A 50 year old male had a syncopal even patient who earlier in the day while standing at church. TRUE statements about syncope include which of the following?

A. Syncope due to an arrhythmia generally is gradual in onset and is associated with a delayed resolution of symptoms after the event.

B. Reflex syncope is primarily manifested by tachycardia and low blood pressure.

C. Triggers of cardiac syncope include micturition and phlebotomy.

D. Autonomic dysfunction due to alcohol use can promote orthostasis.

E. Antihypertensive agents promote orthostasis but opiates do not.

#1
Answer: D

An abrupt onset of symptoms with absence of both **a prodrome and post-event symptoms** (e.g., incontinence, oral trauma, post-ictal confusion) suggests arrhythmia as the etiology of syncope. This includes bradyarrhythmias (e.g. high-grade AV blocks or sick sinus syndrome) or tachyarrhythmias (e.g. supraventricular and ventricular tachycardias). Other types of syncope not associated with arrhythmia are summarized in the following table.

Types of non-arrhythmogenic syncope		
Mechanical	**Vasovagal** (reflex, neurally mediated, or neurocardiogenic)	**Orthostatic (postural)**
Causes include: . Valvular dysfunction . Myocardial dysfunction . Severe heart failure . Hypertrophic cardiomyopathy . Pericardial disease (tamponade) . Vascular etiologies: . Pulmonary embolism . Aortic dissection	This results in a **cardioinhibitory response leading to bradycardia and a vasodepressor response leading to hypotension.** Common triggers include: . Phlebotomy . Micturition . Defication	**Hypotension associated with:** . Change in body position . Dehydration . Autonomic insufficiency (e.g. Parkinson's disease, diabetes mellitus) . Alcohol use . Medications (e.g. antihypertensives, opiates, psychoactive drugs)

. Weiner RB et al. Case 25-2018: A 63 year old man with syncope. NEJM 2018;379:670-80.

#2

You review an echocardiogram report stating that your patient has a left ventricular wall thickness of 25 mm. He has presented with several episodes of syncope. You suspect hypertrophic cardiomyopathy (HCM). TRUE statements about HCM include which of the following?

A. It is inherited in an autosomal recessive pattern.

B. The left ventricular outflow obstructive gradient should increase with hydration or with movement from a standing to a sitting position.

C. Unexplained syncope is a risk factor for sudden death

D. For patients with obstructive HCM leading to congestive heart failure, the only management options that are available are pharmacotherapies.

E. Paroxysmal supraventricular tachycardia is the most common arrhythmia in HCM.

#2
Answer: C

Hypertrophic cardiomyopathy is an autosomal dominant disease and can be diagnosed using ECHO or MRI, both of which will reveal a <u>hypertrophied left ventricle without accompanying dilation</u>. Other cardiac or systemic disease must also be excluded make the diagnosis. HCM is undiagnosed more frequently among women and minorities. Average left ventricular wall thickness is 21 mm; however, massive thickness from 30 to 50 mm does occasionally occur. Obstruction of the left ventricular outflow tract occurs frequently and results in gradients $\geq$ 30 mm Hg. Gradients worsen (increase) in severity when left ventricular volume is reduced due to overall volume depletion (dehydration) or reduced preload (standing up). These circumstances worsen drag across the mitral valve and can result in mitral regurgitation.

Sudden cardiac death can occur in these patients and is more likely in those with historical risk factors such as unexplained syncope or sudden cardiac death in a first-degree relative. Risk factors also include recurrent episodes of non-sustained ventricular tachycardia and the development of left ventricular apical aneurysms. Obstructive HCM can lead to the development of congestive heart failure (CHF) and atrial fibrillation (which is the most common arrhythmia in HCM). These patients are initially managed with pharmacotherapy, but those who continue to progress are candidates for invasive treatments such as myomectomy and percutaneous ablation. Transplant is the first line treatment for patients with non-obstructive HCM.

. Maron BJ. Clinical course and management of hypertrophic cardiomyopathy (HCM). NEJM 2018; 379:655-68.

#3

A 67 year old female is being transferred to a tertiary care center for higher level of care and cardiac catheterization from an outside emergency department. The patient is in cardiogenic shock after earlier complaints of chest pain. At the outside hospital, a bedside echocardiogram demonstrated a severely depressed ejection fraction and apical dilation and hypokinesis. Her ECG did not demonstrate a STEMI; however, she is now intubated and on multiple vasopressors. You are considering takotsubo cardiomyopathy or myocarditis as the diagnoses. TRUE statements about these diagnoses include which of the following?

    A. Patients with myocarditis can present in cardiogenic shock, those with takotsubo cardiomyopathy do not.

    B. Myocarditis may have ST segment depression on ECG, but not elevation.

    C. Patients with myocarditis typically have normal troponin levels

    D. Thyrotoxicosis, subarachnoid hemorrhage, and cocaine abuse can cause secondary takotsubo cardiomyopathy.

    E. Patients with secondary takotsubo cardiomyopathy have a better prognosis than those with primary takotsubo cardiomyopathy.

#3
Answer: D

The differential diagnosis for <u>ventricular apical ballooning</u> includes recurrent apical ballooning syndrome, takotsubo cardiomyopathy, acute myocarditis, cocaine-induced coronary vasoconstriction, coronary vasospasm, and in vivo fibrinolysis after thrombosis. Catecholamine-induced ventricular dysfunction is the cause of both recurrent apical ballooning syndrome and takotsubo cardiomyopathy. Primary takotsubo cardiomyopathy is more common than secondary takotsubo myopathy and is typically triggered by emotional trauma. Primary takotsubo cardiomyopathy often presents as chest pain while secondary takotsubo cardiomyopathy more commonly presents as heart failure or cardiogenic shock, resulting in a worse prognosis. Secondary takotsubo cardiomyopathy is typically caused by diseases of the endocrinologic (e.g. pheochromocytoma or thyrotoxicosis) or neurologic (e.g. subarachnoid hemorrhage or stroke) systems, as well as by the induction of general anesthesia, medications, and illicit drug use.

Acute myocarditis is another important diagnosis to consider in patients with unexplained acute heart failure and can progress to cardiogenic shock. It can be differentiated in the emergency department from takotsubo cardiomyopathy by evidence of infection, ST-segment changes, an elevated troponin level, and left ventricular wall abnormalities. Further inpatient testing may reveal inflammatory cells and interstitial edema on endomyocardial biopsy or a nonsichemic (e.g., no anatomic vascular distribution) contrast enhancement on cardiac MRI.

· Loscalzo J et al. Case 8-2018: A 55-year old woman with shock and labile blood pressure. NEJM 2018; 378:1048-1053.

#4

A 41 year old female with a past medical history of recent miscarriage, family history of connective tissue disease (Ehlers-Danlos), and negative substance abuse history presents with chest pain that sounds typical for acute coronary syndrome, dynamic ECG changes with ST segment depressions in V3-V5, a positive troponin level, and an echocardiogram with an area of hypokinesis in the left ventricular inferolateral wall. TRUE statements about causes of chest pain include which of the following?

A. In patients with myocarditis, the troponin is typically negative on presentation and then gradually rises over a period of days.

B. McConnell's sign is when someone clutches their chest with pressure radiating to the left shoulder.

C. Coronary artery vasospasm causes chest pain more often with exercise than at rest

D. Spontaneous coronary artery dissection from pregnancy my be due to hormonal processes.

E. ST segment depression is the most common ECG finding in takotsubo cardiomyopathy.

#4
Answer D

Patients with myocarditis present with elevated troponins that remain stable or gradually decrease over days. Focal myocarditis should be suspected in patients with chest pain and evidence of acute coronary syndrome in the absence of obstruction on angiography. With a pulmonary embolism, elevated troponins result from right ventricular strain. On echocardiography, apex-sparing hypokinesis of the right ventricle (McConnell's sign) may also be present. In Takotsubo cardiomyopathy, however, echocardiography often shows hyperkinesis of the left ventricle with apical akinesis, accompanied by ST-segment elevations or T-wave inversions. Coronary angiography should be performed to rule out obstruction. Coronary artery vasospasm typically lasts only for 5-10 minutes, causes chest pain at rest, and mimics STEMI on electrocardiography. Sublingual nitroglycerin usually relieves the pain. Conditions with a similar mechanism, such as Raynaud's phenomenon, may also be present.

Coronary-artery dissection accounts for up to one-third of acute coronary syndromes among women less than 50 years of age. Features supportive of this diagnosis include recent history of miscarriage, a family history of connective tissue disease, and a lack of traditional cardiac risk factors. Because many patients are diagnosed in the third trimester or post-partum period, it has been hypothesized that hormones are involved in the underlying etiology of the disease. Cardiac CT angiography should be performed first if coronary-artery dissection is suspected, as invasive angiography could induce or worsen a dissection.

. Tsiaras SV et al. Case 39-2017 - a 41 year old woman with recurrent chest pain. NEJM 2017; 377:2475-2482.

CRITICAL CARE

#5

You prepare to place a central venous catheter in the subclavian vein of a patient that is septic and warrants multiple antibiotics and vasopressors. Which of the following is an absolute or relative contraindicating the cannulation of the subclavian vein?

A. Skin infection overlying the target vein

B. Fracture or suspected fracture of the clavicle or proximal rib

C. Thrombosis of the subclavian vein

D. Coagulopathy

E. All of the above

#5
Answer: E

Though no one site is preferred for central venous access, studies show that subclavian vein cannulation may have a reduced risk of infection and thrombosis when compared to internal jugular and femoral sites. Cellulitis overlying the access site, thrombosis of the vein, and fracture of the proximal ribs or clavicle are contraindications to subclavian vein cannulation. Relative contraindications include coagulopathy, as the site is difficult to compress with direct pressure, moderate-to-end-stage renal disease given the risk of central venous stenosis that would compromise future dialysis access, and presence of apical bullae or severe hypoxemia given the risk of iatrogenic pneumothorax that is associated with the procedure.

The procedure should be performed with the patient's bed in 10-15 degree Trendelenburg for maximal venous engorgement and to decrease risk of air embolism. The ultrasound transducer should be placed just inferior and perpendicular to the mid-portion of the clavicle, and a short-axis image of the subclavian artery, subclavian vein, and clavicle should be obtained. The lung lies just inferior and posterior to these structures.

In addition to pneumothorax, arterial puncture is another serious complication of the procedure. It should be suspected if the syringe returns bright red or pulsatile blood; however, these findings may be obscured if the patient is hypotensive or hypoxemic. If arterial injury is suspected prior to dilation, remove the needle and angiocatheter and apply 10 minutes of firm direct pressure at the site (the problem is that it is realtively incompressible and is thus the reason for relative contraindication in the setting of a coagulopathy) . If arterial dilatation occurred, the large-bore catheter or dilator should not be removed as this could lead to a cerebrovascular accident or hemorrhagic shock. In this case, interventional radiology and/or vascular surgery should be consulted.

Amy Kaji

- Schulman PM et al. Ultrasound-guided cannulation of the subclavian vein. NEJM 2018; 379:e1.

#6

Despite your best efforts at aggressive noninvasive ventilatory and pharmacologic therapies, you have to intubate a 75 year old female given her declining mental status and hypercapnic respiratory failure secondary to COPD. TRUE statements about ventilator management include which of the following?

A. The patient should initially be kept minimally sedated.

B. Elevated peak airway pressures are to be expected and can be tolerated if the plateau pressures remain < 30 cm H2O.

C. The initial respiratory rate should be set at a minimum of 24 to help reverse the hypercapnia.

D. Your goal SpO2 should be 100%.

E. If the flow graph shows breath stacking, then tidal volume should be decreased.

#6
Answer: B.

Intubation should be avoided in patients with obstructive disease (asthma or COPD), if at all possible. Once intubated, the primary goal for the ventilation of patients with obstructive physiology is to allow time to exhale. Deep sedation is typically required during the initial hours of ventilator care. Similar to lung protective strategies, an initial tidal volume of 8 ml/kg based on ideal body weight and inspiratory flow of 60-80 L/minute should be selected. The respiratory rate should be started low at around 8 – 10 breaths/minute and hypercapnia should be permitted. PEEP should be kept at 0 cm H2O or and FiO2 titrated to keep SpO2 $\geq$ 88%. In general, an SpO2 of 100% unnecessarily exposes ventilated patients to excess pressures and hyperoxia. Obstructed patients often have and need high peak pressures to ventilate past the bronchospasm; however, as long as the patient is fully exhaling, the plateau pressure should stay < 30 mmHg If the flow graph shows breath stacking or high plateau pressures, the patient needs more time to exhale and the respiratory rate, not the tidal volume, should be decreased.

. LLSA 2019 article - Weingart SD. Managing initial mechanical ventilation in the emergency department. Ann Emerg Med 2016; 68:614-617.

#7

You have just successfully intubated a septic nursing home resident. TRUE statements about ventilator settings include which of the following?

    A. Initial tidal volume should be 4-5 ml/kg.

    B. Volume assist-control (rather than pressure control) is the preferred mode for the critically ill ED patient.

    C. If the $ETCO_2$ is low, you should lower the respiratory rate.

    D. The peak pressure is more informative in adjusting the ventilator settings than the plateau pressure.

    E. If the plateau pressure is > 30 mm Hg, the tidal volume should be increased by 1 ml/kg.

#7
Answer: B

Volume-assist control prevents patient fatigue and is more widely available on ventilators, making it the preferable ventilator mode in the ED. Tidal volume should start at 8ml/kg based on ideal body weight, with an inspiratory flow rate of 60L/min for most patients. Elevated end tidal CO2 values (above expected PaCO2 goal) should prompt an increase in the respiratory rate. Respiratory rates as high as 30-40 breaths per minute are acceptable. Low ETCO2 measurements, however, can underestimate PaCO2 as a result of other causes such as decreased cardiac output and should not guide respiratory rate management. If FiO2 is greater than 50% and the patient remains hypoxemic, a physiologic shunt should be suspected and PEEP should be increased. Respiratory rate should be decreased if breath stacking is observed.

Plateau pressure measurement every hour and reduction of tidal volume by 1ml/kg when above 30cm H2O (to 4ml/kg total if needed) reduces risk of alveolar injury. Tidal volumes should not be adjusted to achieve PaCO2 goals except in settings of severe metabolic acidosis. Plateau pressure represents alveolar pressure while peak pressure includes pressure exerted by the alveoli, as well as the large airways and ventilator itself.

. LLSA 2016 article - Weingart SD. Managing initial mechanical ventilation in the emergency department. Ann Emerg Med 2016; 68: 614-617.

#8

The clinical trials, SALT-ED and SMART, evaluated normal saline against balanced crystalloids in non-critically and critically ill patients, respectively. TRUE statements about these trials include which of the following?

A. Both were double-blinded and randomized controlled trials.

B. The chloride concentration of saline is lower than that of human plasma.

C. Lactated Ringer's and Plasma-Lyte have identical concentrations of chloride.

D. The trials also compared lactated Ringer's to Plasma-Lyte.

E. Both trials favored the use of balanced crystalloids rather than saline for the composite outcome of death, new renal-replacement therapy and persistent renal dysfunction.

#8
Answer: E

0.9% sodium chloride, or saline, is the most common isotonic crystalloid used in the United States. It has a higher chloride concentration (154 mmol/L) than human plasma (94 to 111 mmol/L) and large volume infusions can cause a hyperchloremic metabolic acidosis and may impair renal perfusion and increase renal inflammation. In contrast, physiologically balanced crystalloids, such as lactated Ringer's solution and Plasma-Lyte, have chloride concentrations that fall closer to the range found in human plasma.

Two recent unblinded trials examined the differences of outcomes in patients given saline versus balanced crystalloids, grouping lactated Ringer's and Plasma-Lyte together. In the SALT-ED trial, use of balanced crystalloids in noncritically ill adults resulted in a lower incidence of the composite income which included death, initiation of renal replacement therapy and prolonged renal dysfunction (NNT = 111). In the SMART trial, use of balanced crystalloids in critically ill adults resulted in an absolute risk reduction of 1.1% (NNT = 94).

  • Self W et al. Balanced crystalloids versus saline in noncritically ill adults. NEJM 2018;378:819-28.

  • Semler MW et al. Balanced crystalloids versus saline in critically ill adults. NEJM 2018;378:829-39.

#9

Your charge nurse notifies you that EMS will be arriving shortly with a critically ill adult patient with a respiratory failure. Which of the following regarding emergent intubation in the critically ill patient is TRUE?

A. A repeat attempt with the same technique by the same provider is recommended when difficulties with intubation arise.

B. A front of neck airway (FONA) procedure requires the use of over 10 pieces of equipment, including forceps, a tracheostomy hook, a tube, and a dilator.

C. For intubation, the head should be tilted up 25-30 degrees when tolerated, and to maximize functional residual capacity (FRC), the patient should be sitting up.

D. The ramped position refers to when the external auditory meatus is level with the nape of the neck.

E. If the cricothyroid membrane is not palpable during a FONA, a horizontal incision should be attempted.

#9
Answer: C

This article emphasizes the "vortex" approach to airway crisis management. It consists of 3 attempts each of oxygenation via supraglottic airway, face-mask ventilation, or tracheal intubation. A fourth intubation attempt by an expert is optional. If intubation attempts fail, which occurs about in about 10-30% of critically ill patients, the airway rescue phase is comprised of attempts at supraglottic airway (SGA) placement with interim attempts at face-mask ventilation. Once SGA placement is successful, progression to an emergency front of neck airway (FONA) can be considered. Indications include aspiration, difficult ventilation, marginal oxygenation, or when fiberoptic guided intubation via the SGA is not possible.

A FONA is indicated if there is clinical deterioration or failure of rescue oxygenation after failed intubation. If possible, patients should be positioned sitting up with head tilted up 25-30 degrees. Ramping (external auditory meatus in line with the sternal notch) helps in obese patients. The only three necessary pieces of equipment are a scalpel, bougie, and cuffed endotracheal tube (size 5-6).

The steps include:

1. Laryngeal handshake to identify the cricothyroid membrane

2. Making a transverse stab incision through the membrane

3. Turning the blade 90 degrees

4. Inserting the bougie along the blade into the trachea

5. Railroading a lubricated cuffed tube into the trachea

6. Inflating the cuff, ventilating, and confirming position

with capnography

7. Securing the tube.

. Higgs A et al. Guidelines for the management of tracheal intubation in critically ill adults. Br J Anesthesia 2018; 120:323-352.

#10

A 52 year old male with end stage renal disease (ESRD) presents with fever, hypotension, and tachycardia. You suspect that the patient has sepsis secondary to pneumonia. TRUE statements about sepsis and septic shock include which of the following?

A. Since he has ESRD, he should not get the 30 ml/kg IV fluid bolus.

B. The Centers for Medicare and Medicaid Services (CMS) have adopted Sepsis-3 and the use of qSOFA score to define severe sepsis.

C. Prehospital IV fluids have been demonstrated to decrease mortality.

D. Lactate can be elevated from hepatic or renal failure.

E. IV hydrocortisone is recommended for all patients with sepsis.

#10
Answer: D

Sepsis-3 defines sepsis as "life-threatening organ dysfunction caused by a poorly regulated host response to infection." Septic shock is defined as "hypotension not responsive to fluid resuscitation," with a requirement of vasopressors for lactate > 2 mmol/L and to maintain a mean arterial pressure (MAP) ≥ 65 mm Hg. This organ dysfunction can be quantified using the sequential organ failure assessment (SOFA) score. A quicker screen, the qSOFA score, was developed for use outside of the ICU. It awards 1 point for each of its three criteria: respiratory rate ≥ 22 breaths per minute, altered mental status, and systolic blood pressure < 100 mm Hg. A qSOFA score ≥ 2 suggests sepsis. Antibiotic administration within the first hour of presentation is recommended.

CMS SEP-1 quality measures, which evaluate institutional compliance with sepsis bundles, have not adopted sepsis-3 definitions and still have a definition for the category of severe sepsis. Using sepsis-3 definitions, mortality from sepsis and septic shock are 10% and 40% respectively. Pneumonia, followed by intra-abdominal and urinary tract infections, are the most common inciting infections. Blood cultures are positive in a minority of cases and show that gram-positive organisms are more commonly isolated, especially for community-acquired infections. Looking only at ICUs, gram-negative organisms with increasing resistance predominate.

Prehospital IV fluid resuscitation has not been associated with decreased mortality. Elevated lactates in sepsis are thought to be due to impaired aerobic metabolism from tissue hypoxia, but can also be secondary to hepatic or renal failure, among other causes. Despite concerns of volume overload in ESRD patients, current evidence supports administration of the same initial IV fluid boluses. Corticosteroids are recommended for patients with septic shock requiring moderate to high dose vasopressors.

- Guirgis F et al. Updates and controversies in the early management of sepsis and septic shock. 2018; 20:10.

ENDOCRINE

#11

You are reviewing the laboratory values for a patient who was brought in by family for lethargy, fatigue, and constipation. The serum calcium is 13.5 mg/dL. TRUE statements about hyperparathyroidism include which of the following?

A. If she has primary hyperparathyroidism, her serum calcium level will be high and parathyroid hormone will be low.

B. Medical management for primary hyperparathyroidism may include medical management with cinacalcet, which will reduce bone loss.

C. Surgery is recommended for patients with hyperparathyroidism who are younger than 50 years old, osteoporotic, have a pathologic fracture, or have impaired renal function.

D. Post-operative complications are common, even when parathyroidectomy is performed by an experienced endocrine surgeon.

E. Surgery corrects the cardiovascular abnormalities associated with hyperparathyroidism.

#11
Answer: C

The vast majority of cases of primary hyperparathyroidism are caused by a single parathyroid adenoma, with factors such as dehydration worsening hypercalcemia and low levels of dietary calcium or serum vitamin D worsening hormone imbalance. Signs and symptoms of hyperparathyroidism include fracture as a result of decreased bone mass, renal colic, constipation, pancreatitis, obtundation, and neuromuscular weakness, with the latter two occurring primarily in cases of severe hypercalcemia. Depression is correlated with hyperparathyroidism but the two have not been conclusively linked. Long term lithium therapy can present as a mimic of the disease.

Hormone levels in primary hyperparathyroidism include inappropriately high levels of PTH, which is not effectively suppressed, and normal levels of 25-hyroxy-vitamin D. A compensatory increase in PTH as a result of low calcium levels (secondary hyperparathyroidism) can be caused by a deficiency of 25-hydroxy-vitamin D, chronic kidney disease, or malabsorptive diseases. Tertiary hyperparathyroidism occurs in end stage renal disease after chronic calcium, phosphate, and vitamin D changes cause parathyroid hyperplasia.

Surgery is the only definitive therapy for hyperparathyroidism. It has very high cure rates. Complications, such as recurrent laryngeal nerve injury and postoperative hypocalcemia, are rare. It is recommended for patients with osteoporosis, kidney stones or renal insufficiency, neuropsychiatric findings, or age < 50 years old. It has no impact on the cardiovascular abnormalities associated with the disease and its efficacy at alleviating cognitive deficits is debated. Pharmacotherapy includes cincalcet, which stimulates calcium receptors leading to negative feedback on PTH release but has no effect on bone loss, and hydrochlorothiazide, which reduces the risk of nephrolithiasis. Since vitamin D and dietary calcium deficiencies can worsen hyperparathyroidism, patients are recommended to maintain adequate serum 25-hydroxyvitamin D levels and dietary calcium intake.

- Insogna KL. Primary hyperparathyroidism. NEJM 2018; 379:1050-1059.

ENT

#12

A 75 year old male presents with tinnitus. Symptoms have persisted for 8 months and occur bilateral. He states that the noise is "like the hum of a car" and that he notices it more at night. On physical exam, his tympanic membranes are clear and there is no mastoid tenderness or deformity. He appears to be hard of hearing in both ears. TRUE statements about tinnitus include which of the following?

A. First-line treatment for tinnitus includes antidepressant medication

B. First-line treatment for tinnitus includes gingko biloba.

C. Hearing loss is a strong risk factor for developing tinnitus.

D. Imaging is indicated in all patients with tinnitus, especially for age > 65 years of age.

E. The prevalence of tinnitus in younger patients has been decreasing over time.

#12
Answer: C

Tinnitus can be subjective or, less commonly, objective, with the latter caused by abnormalities of blood flow or otoacoustic emissions (spontaneous or evoked by cochlear disorders) that can be detected by an external observer. Its estimated prevalence in the adult population is between 10-25%, and it has an increasing prevalence among younger age groups. It can be associated with impaired sleep, depression, and anxiety. Hearing loss is the strongest risk factor for tinnitus. Concomitant symptoms such as vertigo or poor balance suggest a disorder of the inner ear or more central to it (e.g., acoustic neuroma, vestibular migraine, or Meniere's disease). While the volume and quality having little predictive value on its degree of impairment, they can help identify specific causes. Roaring sounds are suggestive of Meniere's disease, whereas rhythmic clicking suggests a disorder of middle ear bones or muscles.

Evaluation for hearing loss and its causes is an important part of the evaluation of tinnitus given that it frequently resolves if hearing loss can be reversed. Imaging is indicated if tinnitus is unilateral, pulsatile, or associated with neurological symptoms. If no reversible cause is identified, cognitive behavioral therapy, acoustic stimulation, and counseling can reduce distress. Medications have not been proven to reduce severity of symptoms; however, many individuals report spontaneous symptom resolution within 5 years.

- Bauer CA. Tinnitus. NEJM 2018; 378:1224-31.

#13

The patient with facial trauma appears to have a nasal septal hematoma. TRUE statements about this entity include which of the following?

A. A septal hematoma is secondary to bleeding from Kiesselbach's plexus.

B. Ischemia of the septal cartilage can lead to necrosis only if the septal hematoma is left untreated for at least 1-2 weeks.

C. While the gauze or nasal tampon is in place, no antibiotic should be prescribed.

D. If packing is placed, then the packing should be left in place for 7 days.

E. The two main types of nasal packing are sterile gauze impregnated with petroleum jelly and the nasal tampon.

#13
Answer: E

Septal hematomas occur with nasal trauma and require prompt attention. They develop when mucosal blood accumulates in a space between the septal cartilage and its overlying perichondrium, causing a separation of the two structures. As a result, the septal cartilage, which obtains its blood supply from the mucosa, can become ischemic and lead to permanent necrosis and a saddle-nose deformity within as few as 3 days. Bleeding from Kiesselbach's plexus is more superficial and only causes epistaxis.

Treatment involves incision and drainage of the hematoma followed by packing to prevent recurrence. Anesthetize the nasal mucosa using a cotton pledget soaked with lidocaine and oxymetazoline. Use a scalpel to make a 5-10 mm incision on the mucosa, aspirate clotted blood using a small suction catheter, and examine the mucosa. Lastly, packing should be placed using a nasal tampon or sterile gauze impregnated with petroleum jelly to prevent development of a seroma or another hematoma. Nasal tampons are easier to place and more comfortable for the patient than gauze packings. Packing should be left in place for 3 days and patients should take prophylactic antibiotics to cover staphylococcal species while packing remains in place.

- Kass J et al. Treatment of hematoma of nasal septum. NEJM 2015; 3722 e28.

GASTROENTEROLOGY

#14

Which of the following statements is TRUE regarding the digital rectal exam (DRE) and the anal canal?

    A. There are no absolute contraindications to performing a DRE.

    B. In adults, the anal canal is 3 to 5 cm and terminates at the anal verge.

    C. DRE can only be performed in the lateral decubitus position.

    D. When documenting the findings of the DRE, the best way is referring to a clock face.

    E. There are 3 anal sphincters.

#14
Answer: B

DRE should be performed on patients who present with anorectal complaints, abdominal pain, or bowel concerns. Anoscopy should be performed if pathology is suspected in the anal canal. Lack of an anus or patient consent for the procedure are absolute contraindications to either exam. DRE can be performed in many positions, including knee-to-chest, lithotomy, standing, or while prone. Documentation of the exam should refer to anatomical locations of the findings as left, right, anterior, or posterior to normal structures. This method of description is less ambiguous than referring to a location in relation to a clock face, which depends on the position of the patient while the exam is performed.

The puborectalis muscle sling at the anorectal junction and the anal verge define the margins of the anal canal, which is about 3 – 5 cm long. The dentate line separates the anal canal into upper and lower parts. The lower portion is innervated by somatic nerve (pain) fibers. Two muscular layers form the anal sphincters, which help maintain continence. The inner layer forms the internal sphincter and provides continuous anal contraction, helping maintain continence between bowel movements. The outer layer forms the external sphincter, which is under voluntary control and helps maintain continence once there is an urge to defecate.

• Rajab TK, Bordeianou LG, von Keudell A, et al. Digital rectal examination and anoscopy. N Engl J Med 2018; 278:e30.

#15

A 57 year old male presents with 2 days of left lower quadrant (LLQ) pain that feels similar to his three prior episodes of diverticulitis that were treated nonoperatively. His exam is notable for a fever, heart rate of 115 bpm, and tenderness to palpation in the LLQ. His WBC is 15,500/l, and a CT scan demonstrates microperforation of the sigmoid, thickening of the sigmoid, and pericolonic fat stranding without free fluid. TRUE statements about the diagnosis and management of this patient include which of the following?

A. Since this is his 4th episode, he is likely to develop more severe illness and complications, such as free perforation.

B. The prevalence of diverticulosis and the incidence of diverticulitis have been decreasing over time.

C. Since he has a "microperforation" on CT, he will need emergent surgery.

D. Evidence does not support the idea that nuts, seeds, or popcorn cause diverticulitis.

E. The patient will need to have a colonoscopy during the hospitalization.

#15
Answer: D

Diverticulosis refers to asymptomatic diverticular disease, whereas diverticulitis occurs when there is inflammation associated with the diverticula. The prevalence of diverticulosis and incidence of diverticulitis have risen over the past century. Low fiber diets, NSAID use, smoking, and physical inactivity are risk factors for diverticulitis. There is no evidence to suggest that nuts or seeds cause diverticulitis.

Depending on patient factors and the severity of disease, diverticulitis may be managed in the outpatient or inpatient settings. Though antibiotics are routinely provided for outpatient management, some limited data from recent trials have called this practice into question. High fever, immunosuppression, leukocytosis, and complicated disease as demonstrated on CT are some of the factors that may indicate the necessity for inpatient management. If medical management of the condition is successful, the patient is at low risk for perforation, requiring an emergent colostomy. Recurrent episodes of diverticulitis are typically similar in severity to the initial episode.

An emergent operation is indicated for sepsis or peritonitis and sigmoid resection with colostomy creation is the safest and most commonly performed procedure. Colonoscopy is recommended for patients with an episode of acute diverticulitis several weeks after resolution of the condition if one has not been performed in the past 2-3 years.

. Young-Fadok TM. Diverticulitis, NEJM 2018; 379:1635-42.

#16

A 36 year old female presents with pruritus and jaundice. TRUE statements about jaundice include which of the following?

A. Jaundice is usually seen when the bilirubin level is greater than 1 mg/dL.

B. Elevation in direct bilirubin suggests hemolysis.

C. Total bilirubin is a sensitive indicator of hepatic dysfunction.

D. Fractionated bilirubin can differentiate hepatocellular injury from cholestasis.

E. Computed tomography (CT) scanning has a similar specificity for detecting common bile duct stones when compared to ultrasound.

#16
Answer: E

Jaundice is not detectable until bilirubin reaches 2.5mg/dL, and it is first noted in the conjunctiva or oral mucous membranes. Quantifying the conjugated and unconjugated components of an elevated bilirubin level helps to determine its etiology. Elevated conjugated bilirubin is suggestive of hepatic dysfunction and a defect in hepatic excretion, while elevated unconjugated bilirubin suggests increased production (e.g., hemolysis), decreased hepatic uptake, or impaired conjugation. Total bilirubin levels are not sensitive indicators of hepatic dysfunction because the liver has a large reserve capacity for metabolizing bilirubin.

A full hepatic panel is needed to differentiate hepatocellular injury from cholestasis as they will have similar fractionated bilirubin levels. An elevation of ALP relative to AST/ALT levels is suggestive of intrahepatic or extrahepatic cholestasis, whereas the reverse is suggestive of a hepatocellular process (an elevating PT/INR in this scenario should raise concern for acute liver failure). CT and ultrasound have similar specificity in identifying common bile duct stones, while ultrasound has superior sensitivity. In the third trimester of pregnancy, acute fatty liver of pregnancy (AFLP), which is characterized by microvesicular hepatosteatosis, presents similarly to HELLP and viral hepatitis.

- Taylor T, Wheatley M. Jaundice in the emergency department: meeting the challenges of diagnosis and treatment. Emergency medicine practice 2018: Vol 20; number 4.

#17

A 2 year old male patient may have ingested an unknown foreign body. TRUE statements about foreign bodies include which of the following?

    A. If an object does not appear on a plain radiograph, then there is no foreign body.

    B. Superficially embedded foreign bodies are best visualized with a lower frequency (3-5 MHz) ultrasound probe.

    C. Animal bones are the most commonly aspirated foreign body by both adult and pediatric patients.

    D. Plastic bread bag clips are typically radiographically visible.

    E. Rectal foreign bodies that are longer than 10cm or sharp are likely to fail removal via the transanal approach.

#17
Answer: E

Not all foreign bodies are radiographically visible. Visibility depends on multiple factors including the objects radiopacity and size, the surrounding anatomic structures, and the patient's body habitus. Higher frequency (7-12 MHz) linear transducer probes are recommended to visualize superficially embedded foreign bodies, whereas lower frequency probes may help with visualizing deeper objects. When ingested, plastics, present a diagnostic challenge because they are invisible on radiographs and CT; yet, they can cause gastrointestinal hemorrhage and bowel perforation. Organic foods are the most commonly ingested objects by adult and pediatric populations, and nuts (especially peanuts) are the most common item found on bronchoscopy of pediatric patients. Patients with rectal foreign bodies are more likely to be male and have a delayed presentation due to embarrassment. Imaging with radiographs should be conducted prior to performing a digital rectal exam. The transanal approach will be successful for a majority of colorectal foreign bodies; however, transanal extraction is more likely to fail for objects that are hard or sharp, longer than 10cm, located in the sigmoid colon, or retained for more than two days.

. LLSA 2018 article -Tseng HT, et al. Imaging foreign bodies: ingested, aspirated, and inserted. Ann Emerg Med 2015:66:570-582.

HEMATOLOGY & ONCOLOGY

#18

You are seeing a patient in whom the CBC is consistent with aplastic anemia. TRUE statements about this disease process include which of the following?

A. Aplastic anemia continues to have a very poor prognosis with no effective therapies.

B. The most frequent cause of aplastic anemia is iatrogenic, such as after cytotoxic chemotherapy.

C. Environmental toxins have not been causally linked to aplastic anemia.

D. Viral infections are not associated with aplastic anemia.

E. There are no genetic predisposing factors that have been identified for aplastic anemia.

#18
Answer: B

Aplastic anemia is characterized by a fatty replacement of hematopoietic stem cells that results in a hypocellular bone marrow. This can be caused by direct damage to marrow from chemical or physical damage that is most commonly due to iatrogenic etiologies, genetic mechanisms, or immune-mediated processes. Iatrogenic etiologies include chemoradiation and toxic exposures such as from industrial benzene use.

Management of the aplastic anemia depends on the underlying etiology. Many patients show recovery of adequate blood counts after treatment with immunosuppressive therapies and require maintenance therapy with a calcineurin inhibitor (e.g., cyclosporine). Bone marrow transplantation is curative. Survival after transplantation from HLA-matched related and unrelated donors is similar; however, serious graft-versus-host disease is twice as likely with unrelated donors. Young patients have better outcomes with transplantation, and children have had success with umbilical cord blood transplantation. Androgens are used for management of constitutional symptoms associated with the condition. Though aplastic anemia does not respond to hematopoietic growth factors, a synthetic version of thrombopietin called eltrombopag has been effective in refractory, severe cases.

. Young NS. Aplastic Anemia. NEJM 2018; 379:1643-56.

#19

TRUE statements about oncologic emergencies include which of the following?

    A. The most common presentation of metastatic spinal cord compression is autonomic dysfunction, such as urinary retention.

    B. In the patient with suspected metastatic spinal cord compression, immediate radiotherapy should be initiated prior to surgery and corticosteroid administration.

    C. The 4 lab tests that one should order to establish tumor lysis syndrome include calcium, phosphorous, potassium, and uric acid.

    D. First line treatment of choice for tumor lysis syndrome is alkalinization of urine.

    E. Treatment of neutropenic fever should include dual therapy for pseudomonas with cefepime and a quinolone.

#19
Answer: C

The most common presenting symptom of metastatic spinal cord compression (MSCC) is back pain. Motor and sensory deficits are the next most common symptoms and autonomic dysfunction occurs late in the disease course and is rarely an isolated symptom. MRI imaging of at least the thoracic and lumbar, if not also cervical, segments should be performed in all patients with suspected MSCC. CT is second line imaging, while plain radiographs should not be used to rule out MSCC as compression can occur without cortical bone involvement. Dexamethasone 10mg IV should be given immediately to patients with suspected MSCC with neurological symptoms to reduce vasogenic edema and mass effect. Patients with more severe and dense deficits should receive dexamethasone. Asymptomatic metastases or isolated back pain can be treated without steroids. Surgery should be performed before radiation therapy in appropriate patients as this improves rates of continence and ambulation.

Tumor lysis syndrome is diagnosed via serum uric acid, potassium, phosphorus, and calcium levels and the presence of at least one clinical feature, such as neurological dysfunction, arrhythmias, or kidney injury requiring hemodialysis. Therapy includes IV administration of 0.9% normal saline to maintain >100 ml/hr (4ml/kg/hr in infants). Hypocalcemia is caused by the hyperphosphatemia, and it should not be treated with calcium as it provides further substrate for calcium phosphate formation, unless it is thought to be causing neurologic dysfunction or arrhythmia.

Patients with an absolute neutrophil count <100 cell/mm^3 are at more than a 50% daily infection risk. Infection in neutropenic fever is commonly due to lung, anorectal, urinary tract or skin infections (e.g. cellulitis, central-line associated).

Fever is defined as any temperature of 38.3°C or sustained temperature of > 38.0 °C for at least 1 hour. Neutropenic fever should be treated with broad spectrum, antipseudomonal beta-lactam monotherapy.

- Wacker D, McCurdy MT. Managing patients with oncologic complications in the emergency department. Emergency Medicine Practice 2018; 20:1.

#20

You are seeing a 39 year old male who has had several months of epistaxis, easy bruising, and generalized fatigue. A CBC demonstrates leukopenia, anemia, and thrombocytopenia. TRUE statements about pancytopenia include which of the following?

A. There is no role for a peripheral smear in distinguishing the etiologies of pancytopenia.

B. Although several nutritional deficiencies and toxins may cause the suppression of one or two cell lines, none cause pancytopenia.

C. Infectious agents can cause bone marrow failure, infiltration, or replacement, leading to pancytopenia.

D. A peripheral smear that demonstrates pancytopenia and reticulocytosis would be consistent with bone marrow failure.

E. Hairy cell leukemia is a common, chronic T cell lymphoproliferative disorder that causes pancytopenia.

#20
Answer: C

Pancytopenia can be the manifestation of many diseases. A peripheral blood smear can be helpful in determining the etiology, especially if immature cells (suggestive of cancer) or evidence of significant hemolysis is present. Other causes include nutritional deficiency, toxins, infection, and autoimmune diseases (drug-induced, systemic lupus erythematosus). Infection can lead to bone marrow suppression (e.g. hepatitis B/C, HIV) or bone marrow infiltration (e.g. fungal or mycobacterial disease) that can result in pancytopenia. Aplastic anemia is often associated with autoimmune pathology that causes bone marrow failure with a peripheral smear demonstrating pancytopenia and reticulocytopenia in the absence of hemolysis or immature cells. Tickborne diseases such as anaplasmosis can cause leukopenia and thrombocytopenia.

Clonal disorders (e.g., myelodysplastic syndrome, acute myeloid leukemia, hairy cell leukemia, and non-Hodgkin's lymphoma) can also cause cytopenias. Hairy cell leukemia is a rare, chronic B cell clonal disorder which presents in middle-aged men with fatigue, bleeding, or infection. Massive splenomegaly and cytopenia, which occurs in nearly all patients due to cytokine-mediated bone marrow suppression, are common.

• Iyasere CA, et al. Case 28-2018: a 39-year old man with epistaxis, pain and erythema of the forearm, and pancytopenia. NEJM 2018; 379:1072-81.

#21

A 32 year old woman presents to the ED with left upper quadrant abdominal pain, severe headache and loss of peripheral vision. Four weeks prior, the patient underwent elective termination of a pregnancy with methotrexate. Conception occurred in the presence of an intrauterine device. which was removed after the termination. Oral contraceptives were initiated afterwards and the patient is a smoker. The patient's abdominal exam is notable for left upper quadrant tenderness to palpation and she has decreased peripheral vision superiorly and inferiorly in the left visual field on neurological exam. Labs are notable for anemia, thrombocytopenia, and an elevated D-dimer. There are no schistocytes seen on peripheral blood smear. CT of the head and neck demonstrates a small, focal area of hyperdensity (consistent with hemorrhagic conversion) and cerebral vein thrombosis. CT of the abdomen demonstrated splenomegaly and splenic vein thrombosis. TRUE statements include which of the following?

A. Microangiopathic hemolytic anemia is defined by the presence of at least 10% of schistocytes per high power field.

B. Anemia with a low lactate dehydrogenase level and an elevated haptoglobin level suggests a hemolytic process.

C. Spherocytes are typically seen in cold agglutinin disease.

D. A negative direct antiglobulin test (Coombs' test) is consistent with warm and cold autoimmune hemolytic anemia.

E. There are two options for treatment of classic

paroxysmal nocturnal hemoglobinuria (PNH), including eclulizumab and allogenic bone marrow transplantation.

#21
Answer E

Microangiopathic hemolytic anemia (MAHA) is a result of mechanical damage of red blood cells and can occur in numerous conditions, including thrombotic thrombocytopenic purpura, hemolytic uremic syndrome, eclampsia, malignant hypertension, vasculitis, and valvular heart disease. The presence of > 1% schistocytes per high-power field on blood smear suggests microangiopathic disease. Anemia, elevated lactate dehydrogenase, and low haptoglobin suggest hemolysis. Additional notable findings include spherocytes, red-cell clumping, and positive Coombs' test, which suggest autoimmune hemolytic anemia, cold agglutinin disease, or warm or cold autoimmune hemolytic anemia, respectively. Urinalysis with blood but no red cells on microscopic analysis suggests intravascular hemolysis resulting in hemoglobinuria without hematuria. Splenomegaly, anemia, and jaundice are characteristic of extravascular hemolysis.

Hemoglobinuria, macrocytosis, thrombocytopenia, and history of thrombotic events raise suspicion for paroxysmal nocturnal hemoglobinuria (PNH), which, paradoxically, does not cause nocturnal symptoms. Many women with PNH receive the diagnosis during pregnancy when it is presumed that the elevated estrogen levels contribute to an increased thrombotic risk.

Hemoglobinura from intravascular hemolysis is thought to trigger smooth-muscle spasm causing abdominal pain in this disorder, while the mechanism of bone marrow dysfunction is less lear. Overall, thrombotic events are the most common cause of death in patients with PNH. Treatment includes eculizumab, which prevents formation of the membrane attack complex and subsequent complement-driven intravascular hemolysis. Bone marrow transplantation is indicated in patients who do not respond to eculizumab, cannot afford it, or who have bone marrow suppression affecting multiple cell lines.

• Sykes DB et al. Case 40-2017 - a 32 yo female with headache, abdominal pain, anemia, and thrombocytopenia. NEJM 2017; 377:2581-2590.

#22
There are now several patients in the ED that are presenting with anemia and "need for blood transfusion." There is the patient who gets transfused weekly at the transfusion center but is in the ED today because the center was closed. Then, there is the patient with a GI bleed, another with sickle cell disease, one with menorrhagia, and a trauma patient! TRUE statements about blood transfusion include which of the following?

A. The shelf life of refrigerated preserved blood in the U.S. is 28 days.

B. There have been several randomized clinical trials that demonstrate that in the setting of acute coronary syndrome, blood should be transfused if the Hb is <10.

C. Voluntary blood donations in the U.S. are tested for syphilis and Chagas' disease.

D. The most common complication of blood transfusion in the U.S. is infection transmission.

E. Massive transfusion can be complicated by hypokalemia and hypocitratemia.

#22
Answer: C

Red cells are kept in preservative solution and have a refrigerated shelf life of up to 42 days. One unit of red blood cells should result in an increase in serum hemoglobin by 1 g/dL and has a volume of 350 mL. Although multiple guidelines for transfusion exist, a hemoglobin of 7-8 g/dL is a common threshold for transfusion in asymptomatic patients. Indications for transfusion in more complex patient populations, including those with acute coronary syndrome, hematologic disorders, long-term dependence on transfusions, cancer, and neurologic disorders are less clear.

Blood donations in the United States are tested for many diseases, including hepatitis B and C, HIV, Chagas disease, syphilis, Zika virus, and others. While detected pathogens can be inactivated in platelets and plasma by existing technology, it is unable to do so in blood. Today, noninfectious complications of blood transfusion are more common than infectious complications. Transfusion associated circulatory overload, which results in a cardiogenic pulmonary edema, is among the most common complications. Other complications include transfusion related acute lung injury (a non-cardiogenic pulmonary edema mediated by antibodies in donor plasma), graft versus host disease (a rare complication with a high mortality that can be prevented by inactivating T cells in the donor blood components by irradiation), and iron overload. Massive transfusion can cause a dilutional coagulopathy, hypothermia, hyperkalemia, and citrate toxicity. Citrate is used as an anticoagulant that binds divalent cations causing hypocalcemia and hypomagnesemia. It is metabolized by the liver to bicarbonate, resulting in a metabolic alkalosis.

• Carson JL et al. Indications for and adverse effects of red cell transfusion. N Engl J Med 2017; 377:1261-72.

INFECTIOUS DISEASE

#23

You are seeing a 35 year old female who presents with fever, headache, and myalgias. Of note is her hemoglobin of 6 g/dL, whereas it was 10 g/dL several weeks prior. In your differential diagnosis, you consider aplastic crisis. TRUE statements about aplastic crisis and parvovirus B19 include which of the following?

    A. Parvovirus B19 typically causes a "slapped cheek" rash in adults who become infected with the virus.

    B. Consequences of infection during pregnancy are greater if the woman is later in gestation (> 20 weeks).

    C. Routine antepartum screening tests for parvovirus.

    D. In children who are infected with parvovirus B19, typical symptoms include cough and coryza.

    E. Anemia and high-output failure can occur in the fetus of a parvovirus B19 infected mother.

#23
Answer: E

Antibody-mediated red cell aplasia can be caused by viral infections, hematologic malignancies, pregnancy, and autoimmune conditions. Acute infection with Parvovirus B19 causes temporary hypoproliferative anemia by infecting erythrocytes and their precursors. Viremia is often prolonged in immunosuppressed patients. Initial symptoms in adults are general and include fever, malaise, and headache. In children, its classic manifestation is known as erythema infectiosum and is characterized by a "slapped cheek" rash.

Routine antepartum screening does not test for parvovirus infection. Maternal infection during pregnancy can lead to intrauterine fetal demise as a result of anemia, high-output failure, and hydrops fetalis. Intrauterine fetal demise is more common in those infected before 20 weeks of gestation. When complications develop, intrauterine red blood cell transfusion may be necessary.

- Knuesel SJ, Guseh S, Karp Lead R, et al. Case 6-2018: a 35 year old woman with headache, subjective fever, and anemia. NEJM 2018; 378:753-760.

#24

A 5 year old male is brought in by paramedics after he was bitten on the head, face, and neck by a pit bull. TRUE statements about mammalian bites include which of the following?

A. A bite on the face should not be closed primarily because of increased infection rates.

B. If the patient returns in five days with cellulitis and a wound infection, it is most likely secondary to Pasteurella.

C. Sepsis is the most common presentation of an infection by Capnocytophagia, particularly in an alcoholic or asplenic patient.

D. Bites by dogs are more prone to infection than those by cats or humans.

E. Pasteurella can cause cat scratch disease.

#24
Answer: C

Dog bites are generally minor; however, fatalities can occur and are typically due to pit bulls and pit bull mixes. While infections from animal bite wounds are commonly polymicrobial, the Pasteurella species is the most frequently isolated organism from infected dog (Pasteurella canis) and cat (Pasteurella multocida and septica) bite wounds. Pasteurella infections present with a localized cellulitis within 24 hours of injury, unlike infections from other pathogens that present 2-3 days later. Capnocytophagia canimorus, found in the oral flora of up to 40% of dogs, can cause a severe infection in alcoholics and patients post-splenectomy. It most commonly presents with sepsis, followed by meningitis, and complications include TTP, DIC, and septic shock.

Puncture animal bite wounds and wounds that are longer than 3 cm are more likely to become infected. Cat bites become infected more frequently than dog bites and can result in the formation of a septic pseudoaneurysm as a result of direct vessel trauma and subsequent bacterial colonization. This presents with pain, swelling, and a pulsatile mass. Dog bites, especially in cosmetically significant areas, should be primarily closed, ideally within 8 hours of injury. Cat scratch disease is caused by Bartonella henselae and is another complication that often self resolves but may require rifampin or trimethoprim/sulfamethoxzole if systemic signs and symptoms occur.

- Aloi MS et al. Mammalian bites. Trauma reports 2018;19:3.

#25

A 42 year old female nurse presents to the ED with fever, headache, and joint pains. She has diabetes, hypertension, and arthritis. She returned from the Dominican Republic five days ago. She is convinced that she has dengue fever. She is febrile and looks uncomfortable. Her fingers, wrists, and ankles are swollen and tender. She has a maculopapular rash. In addition to dengue fever, you consider chikungunya virus (CHIKV), as well as other emerging infectious diseases, such as Zika (ZIKV), and Middle East respiratory syndrome (MERS). TRUE statements about CHIKV, ZIKV and MERS include which of the following?

A. A MERS outbreak has never occurred outside of the Middle East.

B. Patients with CHIKV will typically complain of arthralgias of proximal joints more frequently than of distal joints.

C. Male patients with ZIKV should engage in birth control practices for 6 months or more.

D. The rash exhibited by those with CHIKV is typically pustular.

E. The conjunctivitis associated with ZIKV is typically associated with copious mucopurulent discharge.

#25
Answer: C

MERS, chikungunya (CHIKV), and Zika (ZIKV) are emerging infections, defined as those whose incidence has increased recently or is likely to increase in the future. Emerging infections are typically a consequence of complex, international environmental interactions.

The MERS virus was first identified in Saudi Arabia in 2012 and spreads through zoonotic transmission via the Arabian camel as its animal reservoir. It has a 5-12 day incubation period followed by an influenza like illness that often affects middle-aged persons. As with many worldwide infections, prevention of secondary transmission via early identification and appropriate quarantine are important. A lack of these measures resulted in an outbreak of the disease in South Korea in 2015. Suspected cases should receive PCR testing of nasal secretions or tracheal aspirates. Treatment for MERS is supportive.

CHIKV is an arbovirus that is transmitted by mosquito bites that causes symptoms similar to dengue in travelers and is not uncommonly diagnosed in the United States. It has 3-7 day incubation period, followed by development of high fever and bilateral, symmetric, distal greater than proximal joint arthralgias. A maculopapular, vesicular, or bullous rash in addition to other nonspecific symptoms, such as headache and myalgias, can occur. Common laboratory abnormalities include elevated transaminases, hypocalcemia, lymphopenia, and rarely, thrombocytopenia. PCR testing is diagnostic and sensitive. Treatment for CHIKV is supportive.

ZIKV is a flavivirus that is similar to West Nile, yellow fever, and Japanese encephalitis viruses and is transmitted by mosquitos. It was declared a public health emergency in 2016 due to its association with congenital microcephaly, the risk of which is thought to be greatest with first trimester exposure. The diagnosis can be made clinically in a patient with travel to an endemic area within the past week who presents with a low-grade fever, nonpurulent bilateral conjunctivitis, retro-orbital headache, and a fine, pruritic maculopapular rash that spreads diffusely over the body and has palmoplantar involvement. PCR testing is the diagnostic test of choice. In women planning to become pregnant, additional IgM and confirmatory testing is recommended. Treatment is supportive. Infected women with a negative pregnancy test are advised to use birth control for at least two months and male patients are recommended to use appropriate birth control measures for at least 6 months.

. Millan R et al. Recognizing and managing emerging infectious diseases in the emergency department. Emergency Medicine Practice 2018 vol. 20, number 5.

#26

A 45 year old male patient with newly diagnosed HIV presents for evaluation of a large mass in his liver. Imaging and biopsy confirm that it is hepatocellular cancer, and you wonder whether HIV predisposes to this cancer and whether it is an AIDS-defining illness. TRUE statements about HIV-associated cancers and related diseases include which of the following?

A. Hepatocellular cancer secondary to hepatitis B virus (HBV) or hepatitis C virus (HCV) is an AIDS-defining cancer.

B. Most HIV-associated cancers are caused by dysregulation of immune response by bacteria or fungi.

C. Kaposi's sarcoma associated herpesvirus (KSHV) can be sexually transmitted.

D. Overall survival for patients with HIV-associated lymphoma has unfortunately remained low at 20%.

E. Head and neck cancers are the most common HPV-associated tumors.

#26
Answer: C

AIDS-defining cancers including Kaposi's sarcoma, aggressive B-cell lymphomas, and invasive cervical cancer. Lung cancer, oropharyngeal cancer, hepatocellular and many other types of cancer are more common in patients with HIV but do not define progression to AIDS. HIV-associated cancers are caused by well-established oncoviruses due to HIV-induced immune dysregulation which impairs virus control and leads to development of cancer. Oncogenic viruses can be transmitted by sex (e.g. KSHV, HBV, HPV) or needle-sharing (e.g. HBV, HCV), or can be related to quantifiable immunologic factors, such as CD4 count (e.g. Kaposi's sarcoma). Unfortunately, while manifestations of KSHV can be treated with anti-retroviral therapy, recurrence can occur. HIV-associated lymphomas, of which there are many, have a much-improved survival rate as a result of antiretroviral therapy. HPV-associated cancers, which most commonly affect the cervix or anus, as well as hepatocellular cancer from HBV, can be prevented by vaccination.

. Yarchoan R, Uldreick TS. HIV-associated cancers and related disease. NEJM 2018; 378:1029-41.

#27

A 20 year old male student presents with six days of headache, four days of fever, and one day of neck stiffness, as well as a non-pruritic rash that began on the trunk and spread to his extremities. He lives in southern California, but he returned from a vacation on a cattle ranch in Texas seven days ago where he was exposed to many farm animals. On exam, he is a non-toxic appearing male with a temperature to 39.3° C, heart rate of 75, normal blood pressure, and normal respiratory rate. He has a supple neck and a faint, pink, morbilliform rash on the trunk. Labs demonstrate a mild transaminitis and mild thrombocytopenia. You think the patient may have murine typhus. TRUE statements about murine typhus include which of the following?

A. There have been no known cases of murine typhus in California over the last century.

B. The life cycle of R. Typhi includes a dog-cat-horse-tick sequence.

C. Patients may exhibit a temperature-pulse dissociation with both fever and relative bradycardia.

D. The diagnosis is clinched by a positive stool culture.

E. The treatment of choice is penicillin.

#27
Answer: C

Murine typhus incubates for 5-15 days and presents with non-specific signs and symptoms, which in decreasing order of prevalence include fever (present in > 99% of patients), headache, malaise, and myalgias. The most common exam findings in decreasing order of prevalence include rash (present in about half of patients), hepatomegaly, and splenomegaly. Laboratory findings include elevated transaminases, lactate dehydrogenase, and thrombocytopenia. The triad of fever, headache, and rash is found in less than half of all patients. Temperature-pulse dissociation (fever without tachycardia) can occur in murine typhus, as well as other infections driven by obligate intracellular organisms such as Rocky Mountain spotted fever or medical conditions such as CNS lesions. Severe complications such as respiratory failure, aseptic meningitis, and septic shock may develop, but overall mortality is very low even without antibiotics. Diagnosis can be made by high or increasing indirect immunofluorescence assay titers, which are positive in half patients one week into the illness. PCR testing or microscopic isolation of bacteria can also be used. Empiric treatment should be provided while awaiting diagnostic test results. Doxycycline is first-line and decreases length of illness from two weeks to less than four days. Ciprofloxacin can be used in patients with contraindications to doxycycline.

- Stern RM et al. A headache of a diagnosis. N Engl J Med 2018; 379:475-479.

#28

TRUE statements about patients with HIV/AIDS presenting to the ED include which of the following?

    A. Due to improved screening and testing, 95% of individuals with HIV have received the diagnosis.

    B. Unfortunately, current antiviral medications are poorly tolerated by patients, and nearly two-thirds of patients end up switching regimens.

    C. HIV medications should only be started if the CD4 count is < 500 cells/mm^3.

    D. Post-exposure prophylaxis consists of a standard 3-drug antiretroviral regimen for one month.

    E. The earliest that the new antigen/antibody/immunoassay testing for HIV can detect an acute infection is thirty days after initial exposure.

#28
Answer: D

Nearly 1/5 of individuals with HIV are unaware of their diagnosis and many more do not receive regular care. Recently, it has become clear that early initiation of antiretroviral therapy (regardless of CD4 count) is beneficial. Other indications for antiretroviral therapy include post-exposure prophylaxis and pre-exposure prophylaxis in high risk patients. Drug regimens for post-exposure prophylaxis are the same drug combinations used in patients with HIV and consist of a 1-month course of a standard 3 antiretroviral drug regimen. Post-exposure prophylaxis is provided for occupational exposures, as well as unprotected sexual encounters or exposure to blood of an HIV-infected individual in an IV drug user within 72 hours. Benefits of immediate treatment include reduction in cardiovascular risk and mortality as a result of decreased viral reservoirs and reduction in chronic negative impacts on the immune system. The risk of transmission is increased in acute HIV as a result of high viral load. Pre-exposure prophylaxis is indicated in various populations, including commercial sex workers, HIV-discordant couples, and injection drug users. Before prescribing pre-exposure prophylaxis, a negative HIV test is important to prevent partial treatment of HIV. New HIV antigen-antibody tests can detect HIV 10 days after exposure, while a HIV-1 RNA viral load test may be positive up to 3 days sooner.

- Stanley K, et al. HIV prevention and treatment: the evolving role of the emergency department. Ann Emerg Med 2017; 70: 562-572.

MISCELLANEOUS

#29

There is a prehospital radio call regarding a 22 year old male who has sustained an electrical injury. The medics state that they are on scene with the patient who appears to have been thrown from a significant height after he was holding on to a live wire. He appears to be in cardiac arrest and has signs of extensive cutaneous burns to his hands. They are looking to you for on-line medical direction. TRUE statements about the management of this patient include which of the following?

A. With respect to CPR, since this is an electrical injury, ventilations take priority over circulation.

B. If the patient is still connected to the electrical source, the medics cannot approach the patient.

C. Because the patient has burns to the hands, the patient should be transferred to a burn center, rather than a trauma center.

D. Patients who sustain cardiac arrest from an electrical injury have a poor response to CPR, when compared to arrest from all other etiologies.

E. The extent of the surface burns is consistent with the extent of visceral and muscle damage.

#29
Answer: B

Electrical injuries can be difficult to recognize if there is inadequate history, as presentation may resemble that of a typical burn, trauma or cardiac patient. The most common mechanism of an electrical injury occurs when a patient grasps an electrical source with their hands. If there is sufficient current, tetany may result in an inability to release the grip, orthopedic trauma, or respiratory paralysis.

The extent of surface burns does not correlate well with the extent to which there may be damage to deeper tissues. Alternating current (AC) is found in many household lower-voltage applications and causes more damage to electrically sensitive tissues (e.g. nerve, muscle). High versus low voltage is arbitrarily defined by the threshold of 600V. A vertical pathway of electrical shock through the torso or a large surface burn portend a higher risk myocardial injury.

Scene safety is of utmost importance for first responders who are called to the scene of an electrical exposure. Prehospital personnel should ensure the voltage source has been shut off prior to approaching a patient who is still connected to the source. Standard ACLS guidelines should be followed for these cardiac arrest patients. They have higher success rates of CPR as they are less comorbid than the typical arrest patient. Continuous cardiac monitoring and an EKG should be performed for patients with decreased consciousness or syncope. Patients should be transported to a trauma rather than burn center if significant trauma is suspected.

. Gentges J, Schrieche C. Electrical injuries in the emergency department: an evidence-based review 2018; 20.

#30

The paramedics bring in a patient who has sustained an electrical injury secondary to a lightning strike. TRUE statements about lightning strike injuries include which of the following?

A. If the patient had wet skin, he is protected from deeper injuries, because moisture causes increased resistance to electricity.

B. Lightning strike injuries cannot occur indoors.

C. If the patient has a fine branching rash that resembles bare tree branches, the patient should be treated with 1% hydrocortisone cream.

D. Tympanic membrane rupture is very uncommonly associated with lightning strikes.

E. Keraunoparalysis, which is a temporary condition that mimics spinal cord injury, may occur.

#30
Answer: E

Though lightning strikes produce voltages in the millions, they only produce milliseconds of exposure time, so the overall energy transfer is limited. When the strike occurs outside in the rain, a flashover effect, where the electrical energy just stays on the surface, is common. This is because wet skin has a low resistance (high conductivity). Rapid air expansion from the strike can cause a concussive blast leading to tertiary blast injuries. If current travels through plumbing or wiring, lightning strike injuries can happen indoors.

Flash surface burns, arc burns, and deeper burns are common in lightning injury. Lichtenberg figures are superficial skin changes resembling bare tree branches that resolve without treatment in a few weeks and are pathognomonic for a lightning strike. Ocular injuries, such as cataracts and retinal detachments, are common and more than half of all cases have tympanic membrane rupture. Immediate or delayed CNS dysfunction including spinal cord injury, ischemic stroke, or keraunoparalysis, a transient paralysis, can result.

Lightning strikes are challenging from a neurologic standpoint. The CNS dysfunction can be immediate or delayed, and can include ischemic stroke, spinal cord injury, or keraunoparalysis, a temporary condition that mimics spinal cord injury.

- Gentges J, Schrieche C. Electrical injuries in the emergency department: an evidence-based review 2018; 20.

#31

You are seeing a 25 year old pregnant female and her 5 year old son who have been brought in by paramedics immediately after they sustained thermal burns during a house fire. TRUE statements regarding thermal burn care include which of the following?

A. The American Burn Association recommends IV fluid resuscitation for all adults and children with > 5% total body surface area (TBSA) burns.

B. The preferred method to estimate the total body surface area is the rule of nines.

C. Pregnant burn patients with any level of carboxyhemoglobin (CoHb) indicating exposure to carbon monoxide should receive 100% FiO2.

D. Succinylcholine is contraindicated for use in intubating burn patients.

E. Silver sulfadiazine is the preferred topical antibiotic as this decreases healing time.

#31
Answer: C

Oxygen at 100% FiO2 is the treatment for suspect carbon monoxide toxicity as this shortens the half-life of COHb to about 45 minutes. It should be continued until COHb levels reach < 15%. Maternal COHb levels do not correlate well with those of the fetus. However, animal studies have shown that fetal levels may be up to 15% higher and its half-life more than 3 times longer. Thus, it is important to place pregnant burn patients with any potential carbon monoxide exposure on 100% inhaled oxygen.

The Lund and Browder chart is an age-adjusted map of skin surface by body part and the preferred method to estimate TBSA as the rule of nines consistently provides an overestimation. First degree burns are not counted towards TBSA involvement. Burns with > 20% TBSA involvement produce a massive cytokine-mediated systemic inflammatory response, which causes intravascular volume depletion and can result in multiorgan failure. Therefore, the American Burn Association recommends that children and adults with > 20% TBSA burns should receive IV fluid resuscitation, preferably with lactated Ringer's solution. Succinylcholine is not contraindicated during the first 48 hours after a burn injury. After this acute period, it is not recommended due to increased risk of hyperkalemia from acetylcholine receptor up-regulation. Topical silver sulfadiazine is associated with longer healing times and no longer recommended.

- Tolles J. Emergency Department management of patients with thermal burns. Emergency Medicine Practice 2018; 20:2.

#32

Four patients are brought from a fire with burns and suspected smoke inhalation injuries including carbon monoxide (CO) and cyanide (CN) intoxication. They each have body surface area burns of approximately 20%. TRUE statements about smoke inhalation injury include which of the following?

A. Smoke inhalation injury decreases fluid requirements because of the risk for pulmonary edema.

B. CO inhibits cytochrome oxidase, but CN does not.

C. A normal oxygen saturation does not exclude CO poisoning.

D. Prophylactic antibiotics are useful in preventing infection in burn patients.

E. For patients who have both CO and CN poisoning, first line treatment is sodium thiosulfate.

#32
Answer: C

Smoke inhalational injury results in (1) upper airway thermal injury that can lead to airway obstruction, (2) lower airway and parenchymal disease that causes pulmonary edema and increased fluid requirements, and (3) systemic cellular dysfunction from CO and CN exposure, both of which inhibit cytochrome oxidase. In addition, CO binds strongly to hemoglobin causing the oxygen to get displaced from the hemoglobin, which leads to lower tissue oxygenation. Even though there is less oxygen in the blood, pulse oximetry may read normal or high because it uses a wavelength that is absorbed by both oxyhemoglobin and carboxyhemoglobin. Venous or arterial blood gas and co-oximetry can be used to identify CO exposure. CN toxicity is typically a clinical diagnosis though a lactate > 10 mmol/L is very sensitive and specific for CN intoxication. First line therapy for CN toxicity is hydroxocobalamin. Second line treatment for CN toxicity in presence of CO inhalation is sodium thiosulfate, but is an inferior alternative (because sodium thiosulfate indues methemoglobinemia causing further hypoxemia). Prophylactic antibiotics are not proven to decrease infection in burn patients.

- Otterness K, Ahn C. Emergency department management of smoke inhalation injury in adults. 2019; 20:3.

#33

A 60 year old male patient who fell asleep while smoking a cigarette is brought in by paramedics after the house fire. The patient is presumed to have inhalational injury, in addition to the 75% total body surface area (TBSA) burns that he has sustained. TRUE statements about inhalational injury include which of the following?

A. The presence of inhalation injury mandates intubation.

B. If a plain chest radiograph is done immediately upon arrival, it should demonstrate pulmonary infiltrates consistent with inhalation injury.

C. The fluid requirements are less for those with concomitant inhalation injury.

D. The most reliable method of making the diagnosis of an inhalation injury is by blood gas.

E. Even if the patient is wheezing, neither prophylactic antibiotic nor steroid treatment is advised.

#33
Answer: E

Burn victims who have smoke inhalation injury have a 20% higher mortality than those without smoke inhalation injury. Mortality increases 60% if a secondary pneumonia develops due to smoke inhalation injury. The body produces an extreme systemic inflammatory response to inhalation injury which leads to patients requiring more fluids to be resuscitated. A majority of in-hospital mortality related to inhalation injury is due to sequelae of initial insult, such as infection and pneumonia, rather than the initial injury itself. Inhalation injury is a clinical diagnosis that is determined by the presence of factors such cutaneous burns around the nose and mouth, singed nasal hair, soot in the airway, carbonaceous sputum, hoarseness, wheezing, and stridor. Bronchoscopy and radiography can be useful in assisting with the diagnosis; however, chest radiographs performed at presentation are typically normal and therefore not useful in assisting with diagnosis or severity stratification. There is currently no evidence to support the use of prophylactic glucocorticoids or antibiotics in the setting of burns and inhalational injury.

- LLSA 2019 article - Sheridan RL. Fire-related inhalation injury. NEJM 2016;375:464-9.

#34

You are seeing an 85 year old female with a history of atrial fibrillation and heart failure. She is taking digoxin, spironolactone, and warfarin. Her daughter brings her in because of confusion, nausea, and vomiting. TRUE statements about her diagnosis and management include which of the following?

A. Spironolactone is contraindicated in patients > 65 years old who have a creatinine clearance of < 35 ml per minute.

B. Digoxin is primarily hepatically cleared.

C. Digoxin is nearly 95% bound to albumin.

D. Infections are rarely the cause of delirium in the elderly.

E. The digoxin level can be measured within a day after the digoxin-binding antibody fragments are administered.

#34
Answer: A

Delirium is important to identify as its diagnosis is associated with increased in-hospital mortality and mortality at 1 year after diagnosis. The next most important step is to determine its underlying etiology. Common causes of delirium in older individuals include hypoxia, hypercarbia, infections, and medication side effects.

Spironolactone use is associated with acute kidney injury and neurologic and gastrointestinal symptoms in elderly patients with a creatinine clearance < 35 ml/min. Digoxin toxicity presents with neurological abnormalities including confusion and weakness, visual disturbances, and gastrointestinal symptoms. A reduction in GFR can lead to an increased digoxin level due to its majority renal metabolism. As about 25% of digoxin is bound to albumin, CHF, older age, and renal failure can also increase risk of toxicity by reducing its volume of distribution. If a diagnostic digoxin immunoassay is desired, blood must be drawn prior to the administration of antidote antibody fragments, which prevents an accurate assessment of the digoxin level until all fragments are eliminated from the body. This can take several days in a patient with kidney dysfunction.

- Mattison MLP et al. Case 15-2018: an 83 year old woman with nausea, vomiting, and confusion. NEJM 2018:378:1931-38.

#35

An 85 year old male with a history of dementia hearing impairment is brought in by his son for being agitated at home. On examination, he will not sit still, attempts to hit the nurse and is clearly confused. He thinks that it is 1970 and that he is on a farm. The blood pressure cuff scares him, as he believes that it is a snake. TRUE statements about this patient's delirium include which of the following?

A. Ideally, the patient should be physically restrained so that no pharmacologic agents have to be administered.

B. The first line pharmacologic agent for delirium is a benzodiazepine.

C. If this patient were quiet and subdued, rather than being agitated, this patient cannot have delirium.

D. There are no FDA approved drugs for delirium.

E. Hypoactive delirium is less common than hyperactive delirium.

#35
Answer: D

Delirium is characterized by the acute development of a fluctuating disturbance in awareness and attention. There are two types of delirium, hyperactive and hypoactive. Hypoactive delirium is more common and has a poorer prognosis. Approach to delirium is primarily focused on first diagnosing the underlying cause of delirium and then addressing all reversible and precipitating causes. Precipitating causes include medications, infections, surgery, acute illness, and pain. Though medications are occasionally used in the treatment of delirium, this is an off-label use and there are actually no FDA approved drugs for delirium. Instead non-pharmacologic interventions (de-escalation techniques and sitters) are first line and interventions (restraints and medications) should be avoided when possible. Though physical restraints are occasionally used with the intent of preventing the patient from hurting themselves and others, studies have shown that physical restraints actually cause increased injury. If pharmacologic agents need to be used, the recommendation is to start with low dose antipsychotics which have a more favorable risk-to-benefit ratio than both benzodiazepines and physical restraints. Benzodiazepines should be avoided due to their potential for increasing delirium.

- Marcantonio ER. Delirium in hospitalized older adults. NEJM 2017; 377:1456-66.

#36

A 55 year old female presents with dry eyes, dry mouth, fatigue, and arthralgias. You suspect primary Sjogren's syndrome. Which of the following is TRUE regarding its diagnosis and management?

    A. Unlike other autoimmune diseases, Sjogren's has a male predominance.

    B. The three symptoms of dry mouth and eyes, fatigue, and joint pain is only present in a small minority of the patients (< 30%).

    C. Treatment relies on muscarinic agonists, such as pilocarpine.

    D. Patients with Sjogren's are at decreased risk for B-cell lymphoma.

    E. The treatment of choice for dry eyes in Sjogren's is ocular glucocorticoid drops.

#36
Answer: C

Sjogren's syndrome is a disease that presents with a relatively common set of symptoms including dry mouth and eyes, joint pains, and fatigue. However, the diagnosis remains challenging as these symptoms are nonspecific. It is diagnosed by either serum anti-SSA antibodies or focal lymphocytic sialadenitis on salivary gland biopsy. Primary Sjogren's syndrome is 9 times more common in women than men and has a peak incidence in middle age. The triad of dry mouth, dry eyes, fatigue, and joint pain are present in over 80% of patients with the disease and lead to a major loss in quality of life.

Sjogren's syndrome can be isolated or occur in association with many other autoimmune diseases such as lupus and rheumatoid arthritis. In 30-40% of cases, patients can have systemic manifestations such as primary biliary cirrhosis, bronchiolitis, and interstitial nephritis. Those with Sjogren's syndrome have a 15-20-fold increased risk of B-cell lymphoma. Primary treatment for Sjogren's syndrome includes muscarinic agonists such as pilocarpine. Hydroxychloroquine has been used as an adjunct to treat arthralgias. In severe organ manifestations, immunosuppressive agents, including prednisone and methotrexate, are occasionally used, similar to other autoimmune disease. Ocular glucocorticoid drops are not recommended for the dry eyes, as they can result in increased intra-ocular pressure and corneal damage.

- Mariette X, Criswell LA. Primary Sjogren's Syndrome. NEJM 2018; 378:931-9.

#37

A 65 year old terminally ill patient with metastatic melanoma is brought in by family for dyspnea and altered mental status. He does not appear to have decision-making capacity. TRUE statements about the care of the dyspneic dying patient in the ED include which of the following?

A. The living will provides specific physician orders that can guide the use of interventions, such as oxygen, intubation, medications, etc.

B. The presence of a death rattle correlates with a median survival of 2-3 weeks.

C. If this patient has not designated a surrogate decision maker, the surrogate is determined by the established state legal hierarchy (patient's spouse is typically at the top of list).

D. Opioid administration, when used to treat dyspnea, hastens death.

E. The doses of opioids to administer for the treatment of dyspnea typically are higher than those given for pain management.

#37
Answer: C

Patients can designate their wishes in a variety of legal documents. A living will provides general preferences for end of life care that are typically more vague, whereas a physician order for life sustaining treatment (POLST) contains concrete physician orders that can guide use of interventions such as intubation. When a patient is unable to make decisions for themselves the law specifies who will make that decision. Designated healthcare power of attorneys chosen by the patient take priority, but if one is not designated then the surrogate is determined by a legal hierarchy of decision makers that varies by state.

The presence of a death rattle (the sound created by air traveling over pooled secretions in the posterior pharynx) correlates to a median survival of 23 hours and can be relieved with medications such as glycopyrrolate. Opioids effectively treat symptomatic dyspnea in end of life care <u>without</u> hastening death. Studies have demonstrated that when opioids are administered to target symptomatic relief of dyspnea, changes in arterial oxygenation and carbon dioxide are not observed. Dosing is started at about 1-2 mg IV morphine or 0.2-0.4 mg IV hydromorphone, which are lower than doses typically used for pain. Fans aimed at the face and supplemental oxygen are two major non-pharmacologic modalities for providing dyspnea relief.

- Shreves A, et al. Emergency Department Management of Dyspnea in the Dying patient. Emergency Medicine Practice 2018.

#38

You learn of an active shooter on the premises of the hospital. TRUE statements about an active shooter situation at a health care facility include which of the following?

    A. There have been no active shooter cases in a US hospital where a death has resulted.

    B. All providers should adhere to the plan to "run, hide, fight."

    C. A different set of responses ("secure, preserve, fight") may be considered for the provider who is in the midst of caring for a critically ill patient.

    D. Entry points to patient care areas should only be able to be locked from outside of the patient care area.

    E. The most common preventable cause of death from an active shooter scenario is psychological.

#38
Answer: C

Between the years 2000 to 2011 there have been 154 recorded active shooter incidents across 40 states, resulting in the injury or death of 235 people. The Department of Homeland Security has created a specific set of guidelines to respond to such incidents. "Run, hide, fight" is the standard response for most public institutions. Run away from the event if possible, hide if you are unable to escape, and as a last resort, fight off the shooter.

While this may be appropriate for most public businesses and situations, hospitals provide a unique set of challenges. Hospitals have patients that are often dependent on staff and equipment for survival. In addition, healthcare workers have a moral and ethical duty to protect their patients in all scenarios. Thus, for essential healthcare workers caring for patients unable to run or hide a different response should be considered, "secure, preserve, fight". Secure the location immediately, preserve the life of the patient and oneself, and fight only if necessary. In these cases, all care areas should be locked and secured from the inside. The most common potentially preventable cause of mortality in these scenarios is bleeding. Tourniquets are essential equipment to preserve lives in active shooter situations. Advanced communication and strategizing with regional law enforcement agencies are important parts of the planning process.

- Inaba K et al. Active shooter response at a health care facility. NEJM 2018; 379:583-586.

#39

A 55 year old male with a history of cirrhosis secondary to nonalcoholic steatohepatitis (NASH) and alcohol abuse presents with alcohol withdrawal. TRUE statements about alcohol use in those with underlying chronic liver disease include which of the following?

- A. There is no known safe threshold of alcohol consumption for patients with chronic liver disease, especially those with hepatitis C virus (HCV), obesity, or metabolic syndrome.

- B. Abstinence can reverse the histopathologic changes of cirrhosis secondary to chronic liver disease.

- C. Alcoholic cirrhosis is the number one reason for liver transplantation in the United States.

- D. In those with poor synthetic function, the benzodiazepine of choice should be a long-acting agent, such as chlordiazepoxide.

- E. There are no FDA approved medications to treat alcohol use disorders.

#39
Answer: A.

Alcohol consumption of any quantity is dangerous in those with underlying chronic liver disease. It causes more liver damage in those with HCV infection, increases the risk of hepatocellular carcinoma in those with Hepatitis B virus (HBV), and increases fibrosis for those with NASH. Cirrhosis only develops in 10-20% of those with heavy alcohol use, but co-morbidities such as HCV, diabetes, and obesity are associated with faster progression to cirrhosis. HCV related liver disease is the leading cause of transplantation in the United States, followed by alcohol related liver disease. While abstinence from alcohol can reverse some effects of alcoholic liver disease such as portal hypertension, once steatohepatitis is present, liver disease is no longer totally reversible. Short and intermediate acting benzos are safer for patients with poor synthetic function. Furthermore, lorazepam is eliminated by the kidney so duration of action is more predictable than medications that are hepatically metabolized, such as chlordiazepoxide. There are 3 medications that have been approved by the FDA for alcohol use disorder including naltrexone, disulfiram, and acamporsate. Disulfiram use is contra-indicated in cirrhosis.

- Fuster D et al. Alcohol use in patients with chronic liver disease. NEJM 2018;379:1251-61.

#40
There are various factors influencing the degree to which clinicians engage patients in shared decision making in the ED. Some are patient factors, others are provider factors, and still others are system and health care delivery context factors and the strengths and limitations of the scientific evidence base. All of the following are patient factors, EXCEPT:

A. Perceived medico-legal risk

B. Acuity of illness

C. Decision making capacity

D. Health literacy

E. Socioeconomic and educational status

#40
Answer: A

Acuity of illness, decision making capacity, health literacy and socioeconomic and education status are all patient factors and will vary from one patient to another. Perceived medico-legal risk is a provider factor. Other provider factors include the practitioner's practice patterns developed over time, willingness to engage patients in shared decision making, cognitive load at that moment in time, perceived equipoise of the decision, understanding of the evidence relevant to the decision at hand, and the ability to rapidly recall and succinctly communicate the benefits and trade-offs of the decision from a patient-centered perspective. System and health care delivery factors include the availability of follow up and population responsibility.

- LLSA 2019 reading - Hess EP, et al. Shared decision making (SDM) in the ED: respecting patient autonomy when seconds count. Acad Emerg Med 2015;22:856-864.

#41

TRUE statements about physician burnout include which of the following?

A. One way to mitigate physician burnout is a reward system whereby compensation is purely based on productivity.

B. Studies demonstrate that, at most, 10% of physicians experience burnout in the United States.

C. Engagement is the positive opposite of burnout and is exemplified by dedication, vigor, and absorption in work.

D. Fortunately, physician burnout has not been associated with quality of care or patient safety/satisfaction.

E. The cost of providing physicians with resources to promote self-care outweighs the benefit in mitigating burnout.

#41
Answer: C

Burnout is a syndrome characterized by exhaustion, cynicism, and reduced effectiveness. Studies suggest that professional burnout has a prevalence of at least 50% among US physicians. Engagement is the positive opposite of burnout and is exemplified by dedication, vigor, and absorption in work. Evidence suggests that compensation based purely on productivity increases the risk of physician burnout. To lessen the potential negative effects of productivity-based pay, some systems have incorporated other aspects (patient quality measures, well-being) as part of the formula. Studies indicate that physician burnout impacts patient safety, quality of care, and patient satisfaction. Because of this, hospital administrators and leadership have attempted to mitigate burnout as the benefits far outweighs the costs. Strategies to routinely measure physician well-being as an institutional performance metric should be implemented.

- 2019 LLSA reading list - Shanafelt TD, Noseworthy JH. Executive leadership and physician well-being. Mayo Clinic Proceedings 2017; 92:129-146.

#42

Over the last several weeks, you have noticed that you dread going to work. When you are there, you also note that you are increasingly doubtful about making medical decisions. You find that you are also angry with the patients and the staff. One of your colleagues suspects that you are suffering from physician burnout. TRUE statements about physician burnout include which of the following?

A. Physicians that work on the front lines of access to care are relatively protected against burnout

B. Burnout amongst physicians has been on the rise in the past decade.

C. Burnout and professional satisfaction is the sole responsibility of the individual employee/physician.

D. Burnout has associated with professional but not personal repercussions, such as broken relationships or substance use.

E. Physicians who spend 5% of their professional effort focused on the dimension of work they find most meaningful have a 0% risk of burnout.

#42
Answer: B

Over the past decade in the US, burnout amongst physicians has been increasing and is much higher than in workers of other fields. Physicians from specialties that are on the front lines of access to care, such as family medicine and emergency medicine, are at the highest risk. Physician burnout is associated with professional as well as personal repercussions, such as broken relationships, substance use, and suicide.

Personal satisfaction and burnout are not the sole responsibility of the individual employee, but rather a system issue. There is plenty of evidence to suggest that a physician's practice environment greatly affects whether the physician will burn out or stay engaged. This provides 9 organizational strategies that can help mitigate physician burnout. They range from calls to first acknowledge and measure the problem to providing approaches on how to cultivate community or provide incentives. For example, when physicians spend at least 20% of their professional time on activities they find most meaningful their risk of burnout is considerably lowered.

- LLSA 2019 reading list - Shanafelt TD, Noseworthy JH. Executive leadership and physician well-being: nine organizational strategies to promote engagement and reduce burnout. Mayo Clin Proc 2017; 92: 129-146.

#43

One of your colleagues takes you aside and confides in you that he is feeling burned out and has had thoughts of quitting. The chair of the department has begun to take notice and is taking steps to identify the causes and implement changes to improve the morale in the department. Physician burnout and distress have been demonstrated to be associated with which of the following?

A. Physician turnover

B. Risk of malpractice suits

C. Physician productivity

D. Physician suicide

E. All of the above

#43
Answer: E

Studies show that physician burnout impacts patient safety, quality of care and patient satisfaction. It has strong links to professional work effort/productivity and physician turnover, which can be costly for the health system as well. Physician distress has also been associated with test ordering and physician prescribing habits, risk of a malpractice suit, and patients' adherence to physician recommendations.

Seven different dimensions are identified in this paper as factors that can contribute to burnout: efficiency and resources, workload, work-life integration, flexibility in work schedule, social community at work, meaning found in work, and the alignment of organizational and individual values.

- LLSA 2019 reading list - Shanafelt TD, Noseworthy JH. Executive leadership and physician well-being: nine organizational strategies to promote engagement and reduce burnout. Mayo Clin Proc 2017; 92: 129-146.

NEUROLOGY

#44

Your patient has a recurrent migraine headache. She is a 35 year old female who has complaints of severe pain with brushing her hair. TRUE statements about migraine headache include which of the following?

A. Allodynia, which is an alteration of nociception that typically causes non-noxious stimuli (e.g. brushing one's hair) to be painful, develops as acute migraine duration increases.

B. Migraine is believed to be a vascular headache.

C. The diagnosis of migraine headache is made based on the characteristic findings seen on MRI/MRA of the brain.

D. First line therapy for migraine headache includes opioids.

E. A minority of ED patients have recurrence of the headache 24 hours after discharge.

#44
Answer: A

Migraine headaches are chronic recurrent headaches that commonly have symptoms such as photophobia and nausea, though there is significant variability in presentation. Symptoms may include allodynia, when non-noxious stimuli (e.g. brushing one's hair) are perceived as painful. Allodynia develops as migraine duration increases. Migraine was once thought to have a vascular etiology given its pulsating nature, but recent evidence from advanced imaging studies has clearly refuted this thought and indicates that it is a disorder of nociceptive processing. Migraine is a clinical diagnosis. There are currently no laboratory or imaging findings available to confirm this diagnosis.

First line treatment for migraines is antidopaminergic medication which work both to relieve pain as well as nausea. Opioids are less successful in migraine treatment. Though antidopaminergic medications are very successful in stopping a headache, two thirds of ED patients with migraine have a recurrence of headache symptoms within 24 hours of discharge. IV dexamethasone has been shown to have some benefit in decreasing recurrence of moderate to severe headaches within 72 hours.

- Friedman BW. Managing migraine. Ann Emerg Med 2017; 69; 2: 202-207.

#45

A 29 year old female with a history of migraine headaches reports severe headache, nausea, vomiting, consistent with her migraine headache exacerbations. TRUE statement regarding migraine headaches include which of the following?

A. Response to therapy can reliably exclude a malignant cause of headache.

B. Laboratory testing, such as CRP is confirmatory for the diagnosis of migraine.

C. The triptans are antidopaminergic agents.

D. Metoclopramide is the first-line agent for migraine headache if her pregnancy test is positive.

E. Akathisia is the least common extrapyramidal symptom associated with antidopaminergics.

#45
Answer: D

Auras are temporary neurologic phenomena characterized typically by visual or sensory symptoms, though they sometimes involve speech or motor function, that precede the headache. As migraine is a clinical diagnosis, routine lab work aside from a pregnancy test, should not be obtained and are unlikely to alter management. Patients may be able to better contextualize their headache amongst their previous headaches once their pain is controlled; however, response to treatment should not be used to exclude a serious cause of headache.

The triptans, antidopaminergics, and nonsteroidal anti-inflammatory drugs have emerged as first-line treatments for acute migraine. The triptans are serotonin agonists and are commonly used for outpatient management of migraine. They several adverse effects, including flushing, chest symptoms, and recurrence. Metoclopramide is an antidopaminergic agent and should be the first line parenteral agent used for migraine patients who are pregnant due to its favorable pregnancy rating. The most common adverse effects associated with antidopaminergic agents is akathisia, which is more prevalent with prochlorperazine than with metoclopramide. Akathisia can be prevented with slower medication administration and treated with diphenhydramine. Ketorolac is the most common parenteral medication used to treat migraine in US emergency departments.

• LLSA 2019 article – Friedman BW. Managing migraine. Ann Emerg Med 2017;69:202-207.

#46

You are seeing a 3-year old male who is brought in by family for 2 days of progressive abnormal language function, lethargy, aggressiveness, spells of unprovoked laughter, athetoid hand movements and orofacial dyskinesias. The boy has no significant past medical history and is fully vaccinated. Of note, he was seen at an outside hospital for a first-time afebrile generalized tonic-clonic seizure 5 days ago. However, because he had vomiting and diarrhea in the days preceding the seizure, he was thought to have an "afebrile, febrile seizure" and did not undergo an LP, EEG, or imaging at the time. Today, on examination, the patient is quiet with a flat affect and subdued behavior. Vital signs are normal, and the patient follows some commands but falls asleep during the examination. He has unintelligible speech and has unprovoked episodes of agitation and screaming. The remainder of the examination was normal. You suspect an encephalitis. Which of the following is TRUE regarding encephalitis?

A. The diagnosis of encephalitis can be made if a patient presents with 8 hours of altered mental status.

B. In the California Encephalitis Project (CEP), anti-NMDA receptor antibodies were identified as a common cause of encephalitis in patients younger than 30.

C. Serum testing for anti-NMDA receptor antibodies is 100% sensitive for anti-NMDA receptor encephalitis.

D. MRI will be abnormal in all cases of anti-NMDA receptor encephalitis.

E. First-line treatment for anti-NMDA receptor encephalitis includes antibiotics and antiviral medications.

#46
Answer: B

The criteria for the diagnosis of encephalitis include the presence of encephalopathy (personality change, lethargy, or an altered level of consciousness) that lasts for at least 24 hours in addition to a seizure, fever, focal neurologic exam, pleocytosis on CSF analysis, or EEG or neuroimaging findings consistent with encephalitis. Based on data from the CEP, anti-NMDA receptor antibodies were the most commonly identified etiology of encephalitis in patients younger than 30.

The onset of anti-NMDA receptor encephalitis is acute though symptoms vary by age. Children less than 12 years old are more likely to experience movement disorders, which are rarely observed in adults. Adults experience seizures, behavioral changes, cognitive dysfunction, and memory problems. CSF testing is the gold standard and is 100% sensitive for anti-NMDA receptor antibodies whereas serum testing for anti-NMDA receptor antibodies is only 85% sensitive. MRI of the brain is normal in half of patients.

Intravenous glucocorticoids, intravenous immunoglobulin (IVIG), and plasma exchange are first-line therapies for anti-NMDA receptor encephalitis. Surgical resection is also considered if a tumor is identified.

- Gorman MP et al. Case 27-2018: a 3 year old boy with seizures. NEJM 2018; 379:870-878.

#47

A 55 year old male patient presents with bilateral hand tremor. The patient does not drink alcohol and does not have a history of alcohol withdrawal. You consider the diagnosis of essential tremor. Which of the following would be <u>inconsistent</u> with diagnosis and treatment?

A. Isolated tremor of both upper limbs

B. Severe dystonic posturing

C. Normal thyroid, liver, and kidney function

D. First-line treatment is propranolol or primidone

E. Bimodal distribution with age peaks in the 2nd and 6th decade

#47
Answer: B

Essential tremor is a syndrome defined by an isolated action tremor of both upper limbs with or without tremor in other locations such as head, lower limbs, or larynx that has been present for at least three years. The tremor occurs as the only neurologic finding and without other neurologic abnormalities such as dystonia, parkinsonism, or ataxia. Essential tremor is a clinical diagnosis based on history and physical; its age of onset has a bimodal distribution in the second and sixth decades. Physiologic tremor occurs at the same tremor frequency but worsens with certain medications, stimulants such as caffeine, stress, or cold weather. These conditions can be further differentiated with basic labs to rule out etiologies that can cause worsening physiologic tremor such as abnormalities in thyroid, liver, or kidney function. First-line treatment for essential tremor is primarily with propranolol or primidone. Refractory cases may require a deep brain stimulator or other interventional treatment approaches.

. Haubenberger D, Hallett M. Essential tremor. NEJM 2018; 378:1802-10.

#48

A 35 year old female is brought in by paramedics after she had a witnessed generalized tonic-clonic seizure. She is no longer post-ictal, and she has never had a seizure before. TRUE statements about new onset seizure in this patient include which of the following?

A. Obtaining an MRI in the emergency department is mandatory.

B. Obtaining an EEG in the emergency department is mandatory.

C. A prolactin level should be ordered to distinguish a seizure from syncope or a pseudoseizure.

D. All antiepileptics medications can cause a rash, ranging from mild maculopapular rashes to Stevens-Johnsons Syndrome (SJS) and toxic epidermal necrolysis (TEN).

E. Oral contraceptives are considered the best method of contraception in patients using anti-epileptics.

#48
Answer: D

When evaluating a patient with new onset seizure, the first step is to rule out other seizure mimics such as syncope and transient ischemic attack. Next, a thorough history should be performed to identify factors such as infection that can lower the seizure threshold and a physical exam looking for focal neurological deficits. Neuroimaging should be done emergently in the setting of trauma, prolonged headache, neurological deficits, or persistent altered mental status. Typically head CT is the first line neuroimaging recommended for all new onset seizures. CT scans do miss some lesions; thus, MRI should be pursued in cases where there is persistent concern for focal abnormality. EEG should be performed emergently if the patient does not return to baseline within 30-60 minutes of seizure activity or has waxing and waning mental status to rule out subclinical seizures. Most patients who return to baseline can have an EEG done as an outpatient to assess the risk of seizure recurrence. Laboratory testing does not typically include prolactin levels since it must be compared to a baseline to be accurately interpreted and can also be elevated in the setting of syncope.

For most first-time seizures without a focal cause, antiepileptic medications are not started. Antiepileptic medications have a broad range of side effects ranging from mild rashes to SJS and TEN. Many antiepileptic medications increase clearance of oral contraceptives, so other birth control methods such as IUDs are preferred for those on antiepileptic medications.

• LLSA 2019 article - Gavvala JR, Schuele SU. New onset seizure in adults and adolescents - a review. JAMA 2016; 316:2657-2668.

#49

A 25 year old male is brought in by paramedics after his friends witnessed a generalized tonic-clonic seizure. The patient does NOT carry a diagnosis of seizure disorder, and this was his first episode. TRUE statements about new onset seizure in adults and adolescents include which of the following?

A. 8-10% of the population will experience a seizure during their lifetime and over half of those people will go on to develop epilepsy.

B. An epilepsy protocol-specific MRI exists, and it includes thin-cut coronal slices to determine risk of recurrence.

C. The presence of hippocampal sclerosis and focal cortical dysplasia does not increase the risk of recurrence.

D. Most states allow noncommercial driving after the first unprovoked seizure.

E. There is no increase in the incidence of sudden death in patients with epilepsy.

#49
Answer: B

Seizures are a common cause of ED visits and as much as 10% of the population will experience a seizure during their lifetime. Despite this high number, only 2-3% of individuals will go on to develop epilepsy. Previously, epilepsy was defined as having 2 or more unprovoked seizures more than 24 hours apart. However, now due to better detection modalities, the definition has changed to include one unprovoked seizure and increased risk of recurrent seizure (at least 60%) in the next 10 years. This increased risk is determined by EEG or epilepsy protocol specific MRI. The epilepsy protocol has increased sensitivity for detecting focal cortical dysplasia and hippocampal sclerosis which, when present, establish the diagnosis of epilepsy. Accurate diagnosis and treatment of epilepsy is crucial as those with epilepsy have a 20-fold higher incidence of sudden death compared to the general public. This is thought to occur due to centrally-mediated severe alterations in cardiac and respiratory function early in the post-ictal period. Though laws vary by state, most states require patients to be seizure free for 6 months after an unprovoked seizure and 3 months after a provoked seizure before returning to noncommercial driving.

- LLSA 2019 article - Gavvala JR, Schuele SU. New-onset seizure in adults and adolescents - a review. JAMA 2016; 316:2657-2668.

#50

A 43 year old male with no known medical history is brought in by paramedics after his friend witnessed him having a seizure that was generalized for 2 minutes. He has never had a seizure before, and he denies any alcohol or drug abuse. He is back to his baseline mental status after approximately 5 minutes. TRUE statements regarding new onset seizure include which of the following?

A. Adults with first time seizure are not at an increased risk for seizure recurrence.

B. Persons with epilepsy are not at increased risk for drowning.

C. Lateral tongue bites are over 70% sensitive for epileptic seizures.

D. Aside from psychiatric medications, no other commonly prescribed medications reduce seizure threshold.

E. Most new users of antiepileptics who develop TEN or SJS develop symptoms within the first 60 days of therapy.

#50
Answer: E

Adults with new-onset seizure have about a 35% risk of having another seizure within 5 years and this risk increases to 75% if they have a second seizure. Persons with epilepsy are more than 15 times more likely to die from drowning than the general public. They should be counseled to avoid high-risk activities such as working at heights, swimming unobserved, and taking tub baths. Lateral tongue bites can help differentiate between epileptic and psychogenic non-epileptic seizures as they are not seen with the latter condition, but are only seen in about 22% of epileptic seizures. Patients presenting with seizure should have their medication lists reviewed as several common medications such as fluoroquinolones, cephalosporins, tramadol, and other psychiatric medications can reduce the seizure threshold. When new users of antiepileptics develop TEN or SJS, more than 90% of them develop symptoms within the first 60 days of therapy.

- LLSA 2019 article - Gavvala JR, Schuele SU. New-onset seizure in adults and adolescents. JAMA 2016; 316:2657-2668.

#51

A 62 year old male with a history of diabetes and hypertension presents with 10 minutes of left arm weakness associated with dysarthria. You suspect that he has had a (transient ischemic attack) TIA. According to the ACEP Clinical Policy on TIA, which of the following is TRUE?

A. In general, TIAs last longer than 2-3 hours.

B. Though the risk of acute ischemic stroke is increased after a TIA, less than 2% of ischemic strokes are preceded by TIA.

C. The risk of delaying neuroimaging in the ED has been quantified as a 50% risk of missing a large vessel occlusive stroke.

D. Current evidence shows that point-of-care carotid ultrasonography performed by an emergency provider is as accurate as MRA and CTA for detecting carotid stenosis.

E. Carotid endarterectomy for severe carotid stenosis performed within 2 weeks of a TIA or stroke significantly reduces future stroke and death.

#51
Answer: E

Historically, the definition of TIA had been based solely on the duration of symptoms; however, in 2009, it was changed to a tissue-based diagnosis that depends on the presence or lack of infarction on imaging. For cases where imaging is unavailable, symptoms lasting more than 24 hours are classified as strokes. Most TIAs last fewer than 1-2 hours.

Patients with TIA have a risk of 3.5% to 10% of acute ischemic stroke within two days, and these percentages increase as time goes on. About 15% of all strokes are preceded by TIA, underscoring the importance of timely evaluations for modifiable risk factors such as atrial fibrillation and carotid stenosis. Carotid endarterectomy for severe carotid stenosis performed within 2 weeks of a TIA or stroke prevents future stroke and death with a number need to treat of 6.

ED workup typically includes at least an initial non-contrast head CT to evaluate for serious alternate diagnoses, though the risk of delaying neuroimaging in the ED is unknown. Carotid ultrasonography is an acceptable form of cervical vascular imaging to help identify high-risk TIA patients; however, currently, there is not enough literature to support the efficacy of point-of-care imaging.

- LLSA 2019 article – Lo, BM et al. Clinical Policy: Critical issues in the evaluation of adult patients with suspected TIA in the ED. Ann Emerg Med 2016;68:354-370.

#52

You are now seeing a 55 year old male who presents with right sided leg weakness associated with slurred speech and a facial droop that lasted 5 minutes but has since resolved. You diagnose a transient ischemic attack (TIA). TRUE statements about TIA, according to the American College of Emergency Physicians (ACEP) Clinical Policy on TIA include which of the following?

A. You can rely upon the ABCD2 score to identify TIA patients that can be safely discharged from the emergency department.

B. There is sound evidence that it is safe to delay neuroimaging from the initial ED workup.

C. In adult patients with suspected TIA, carotid ultrasonography may be used to exclude severe carotid stenosis because its accuracy is comparable to that of MRA or CTA.

D. Even in patients with high-risk conditions (abnormal head CT, suspected embolic source, known carotid stenosis, previous large stroke, and crescendo TIA), a rapid ED-based diagnostic protocol is equivalent to mandatory admission in terms of patient safety.

E. Unfortunately, implementation of an ED-based diagnostic protocol is <u>not</u> associated with decreased hospital costs and length of stay compared with inpatient management.

#52
Answer: C

According to the ACEP clinical policy, risk stratification instruments such as the ABCD2 score cannot be used to safely discharge TIA patients from the hospital. This is because the <u>ABCD2 score does not sufficiently identify patients at high short-term risk of stroke</u>. Head CT can be used as an adjunct to rule out stroke mimics such as intracranial bleeds or masses, but non-contrast head CT alone is not sufficient to determine who is at high short-term risk of stroke. As such, it is unknown if it is safe to delay neuroimaging from the initial ED workup. ACEP recommends that attempts should be made to obtain an MRI as well as cervical vascular imaging such as carotid ultrasound, CTA, or MRA (the three are equivalent). These imaging studies can be used to determine which patients are at short term risk of stroke. Patients with high risk conditions should be admitted to the hospital for stroke evaluation. However, in those without high risk conditions, a rapid ED diagnostic protocol is equivalent in terms of patient safety and has been shown to decrease hospital cost and length of stay. A rapid ED diagnostic protocol includes clinical exams, MRI with diffusion weighted imaging, carotid imaging, telemetry, echocardiography, possible cardiology or neurology consult, and starting anti-platelet agents when appropriate.

- LLSA 2019 article – Lo, BM et al. Clinical policy: critical issues in the evaluation of adult patients with suspected TIA in the ED. Ann Emerg Med 2016;68:354-370.

#53

A 68 year old female with a history of hypertension is brought in by paramedics after she became acutely altered. Her blood pressure in the field was 230/150. Her exam is notable for a dense left hemiparesis and slurred speech. TRUE statements about intracranial hemorrhage (ICH) include which of the following?

A. The blood pressure should not be lowered, since cerebral perfusion pressure should be maintained.

B. A head CT is not necessary because one can distinguish a hemorrhagic from ischemic stroke by clinical scoring systems.

C. Recombinant activated factor VIIa (rFVIIa) is the reversal agent of choice for those with vitamin K antagonist-associated ICH.

D. Prophylactic seizure medication is not recommended.

E. Risk factors for recurrent ICH include younger age and location of the bleed in the basal ganglia.

#53
Answer: D

Intracranial hemorrhage is a true medical emergency and requires rapid assessment and treatment. Initial evaluation should include use of a standardized severity score such as the National Institute of Health Stroke Scale (NIHSS) score. This helps facilitate communication between providers but does not differentiate between ischemic and hemorrhagic stroke. Once ICH is identified on CT or MRI, the focus should be on rapid blood pressure control and reversal of anticoagulation. For those taking vitamin K antagonists such as warfarin, recommended treatment includes vitamin K and prothrombin complex concentrate (PCC). Although rFVIIa can rapidly lower INR, it does not actually replace the clotting factors or restore clotting and is not recommended for warfarin reversal.

High blood pressure is associated with hematoma expansion. In those without contraindications, acute lowering to a systolic blood pressure of 140 is both safe and may lead to improved functional outcomes.

Although anticonvulsant medication is recommended for active seizures and seizure activity on EEG, prophylactic anticonvulsant medication is not recommended. Multiple studies have shown increased death and disability with prophylactic anticonvulsant use and there is no strong association between clinical seizures and neurologic outcome; therefore, they are not helpful and could potentially be harmful. Recurrent ICH is more common in the elderly, and in those with a lobar location of ICH, persistent hypertension, and anticoagulant use.

. LLSA 2018 article - Hemphill JC et al. Guidelines for the management of spontaneous intracerebral hemorrhage. Stroke 2015; 46:2032-2060.

OBSTETRICS AND GYNECOLOGY

#54

A 29 year old G1P0 patient at 9 weeks' gestation presents with intractable nausea and vomiting. Which of the following treatments has <u>not</u> been found to be of benefit, when compared to placebo?

A. Ginger

B. Ondansetron

C. Pyridoxine-doxylamine

D. Antihistamines

E. Acupuncture

#54
Answer: E

While simple nausea and vomiting is common in pregnancy and experienced by most women, hyperemesis gravidarum is a much more severe form that affects less than 5% of pregnant women and is characterized by intractable vomiting, leading to weight loss, dehydration, hypokalemia and ketosis. There is evidence supporting the use of ginger, ondansetron, and pyridoxine-doxylamine in the treatment of nausea and vomiting in pregnancy as compared to placebo. In contrast, there is no significant evidence in support of acupuncture. For mild symptoms the recommendation is to try interventions such as ginger, pyridoxine (vitamin B6), metoclopramide, and antihistamines. For moderate symptoms, pyridoxine-doxylamine, promethazine, and metoclopramide were beneficial.

. LLSA 2019 article - McParlin C et al. Treatments for hyperemesis gravidarum and nausea and vomiting in pregnancy - a systematic review. JAMA 2016; 316:1392-1401.

#55

Your patient is 25 years old and is 12 weeks pregnant. Her urine ketones are 4+ and she has had several bouts of emesis over the course of the week, such that she is losing weight during her pregnancy. TRUE statements about hyperemesis gravidarum and nausea and vomiting during pregnancy include which of the following?

A. Transdermal clonidine is an established treatment for nausea and vomiting in pregnancy.

B. The symptoms of hyperemesis gravidarum usually subside before 20 weeks' gestation.

C. Steroids are recommended in mild cases of hyperemesis gravidarum.

D. The recommendations for anti-emetic use in hyperemesis gravidarum is based on high quality evidence.

E. Ondansetron causes more drowsiness and dry mouth when compared to metoclopramide.

#55
Answer: B

Hyperemesis gravidarum is a severe form of nausea and vomiting of pregnancy that leads to electrolyte imbalances, ketosis, dehydration and weight loss. In some cases, this can even require hospital admission and parental feeding tubes. Symptoms develop in the first trimester around week 6-8 and can continue into the second trimester, but resolving before week 20. For severe symptoms, corticosteroids may be associated with some benefit, though due to potential risks of fetal complications, they should be given only in severe cases. Ondansetron was associated with improvement in symptoms for all levels of severity. Metoclopramide causes more drowsiness and dry mouth when compared to ondansetron. There is one clinical trial with limited evidence supporting transdermal clonidine patches for hyperemesis gravidarum, but given the lack of substantial evidence, it is not an established treatment or a recommended option. Overall, the quality of evidence supporting the recommendations for treatment of hyperemesis gravidarum is poor and based on limited studies with high levels of bias.

• McParlin C et al. Treatments for hyperemesis gravidarum and nausea and vomiting in pregnancy. A systematic review. JAMA 2016; 316:1392-1401.

#56

A 24 year old female G1P0 with an estimated gestational age of 12 weeks presents with intractable nausea and vomiting. She has lost 5 pounds over the last week and has not been able to tolerate anything by mouth. Her urine ketones are positive and she appears to be dehydrated. You suspect hyperemesis gravidarum. Which of the following statements about the condition and its management are TRUE:

A. Outpatient, day-care management of patients with moderate symptoms leads to worse outcomes when compared to inpatient care.

B. Hyperemesis gravidarum is not associated with preterm delivery and small-for-gestational age infants.

C. Oral administration of ondansetron is more likely to cause QT prolongation than IV administration

D. Hyperemesis gravidarum is associated with congenital anomalies and perinatal death.

E. Renal impairment and Wernicke encephalopathy are serious complications that may be prevented by treating the condition.

#56
Answer E

Studies have shown that outpatient management of patients with moderate-severe symptoms is acceptable and results in equivalent outcomes when compared with inpatient therapy. Ondansetron should be used carefully in patients with hyperemesis as their electrolyte disturbances may put them at increased risk for QT prolongation. Intravenous doses of ondansetron larger than 8mg can cause QT prolongation. Oral ondansetron administration has not been shown to cause QT prolongation in adults.

Treatment of hyperemesis gravidarum is important to alleviate symptoms and prevent maternal and fetal morbidity. Maternal complications include extreme weight loss, renal impairment, and Wernicke's encephalopathy. Additionally, hyperemesis has been associated with preterm delivery and small-for-gestational age infants; however, no associations with congenital anomalies or perinatal death have been observed.

• LLSA 2019 Article - McParlin C, O'Donnell A, Robson SC, et al. Treatments for hyperemesis gravidarum and nausea and vomiting in pregnancy. JAMA 2016;316:1392-1401.

OPHTHALMOLOGY

#57

Your patient sustained eye trauma. Which of the following statements is TRUE regarding ocular trauma?

A. Atraumatic periorbital ecchymosis is always benign.

B. If you see fat when you are suturing a lid laceration, it is likely because the patient is obese and has fatty eye lids.

C. Orbital compartment syndrome is best diagnosed by imaging studies.

D. A corneal ulcer appears as a white patch that is visible without fluorescein staining.

E. Pain in the affected eye when light is shone in the unaffected eye is indicative of globe rupture.

#57
Answer: D

When assessing eye trauma, one of the most important components is obtaining a visual acuity. This should only be delayed for irrigation in the case of chemical exposures. Atraumatic periorbital ecchymosis can arise from benign events such as sneezing but can also be caused by a malignancy such as neuroblastoma in children, multiple myeloma, or clotting dysfunction. There is no subcutaneous fat in the eyelids. If fat is visible in an eyelid laceration this is indicative of an orbital septal laceration and there is a high risk of globe penetration.

Orbital compartment syndrome in trauma is frequently secondary to hemorrhage in the orbit resulting in retrobulbar hematoma. Orbital compartment syndrome is a clinical diagnosis based on elevated intraocular pressures, decreased vision, proptosis, and limited extraocular movements. It can lead to ischemia of the retina and optic nerve and requires emergent decompression with a lateral canthotomy. The most important risk factor for corneal ulcer is contact lens use. A corneal ulcer appears as a white patch that is visible without fluorescein staining. Consensual photophobia is pain in the affected eye when light is shone in the unaffected eye. The pain stems from the contraction of the ciliary muscle and is indicative of uveitis.

- Wendell L et al. Ocular trauma. Trauma reports 2018; 19;6.

ORTHOPEDICS

#58

A 2 year old child is brought in by parents because she is not using her right arm and cries when they touch it. The parents believe that it started after the child was pulled by both arms up to stand and walk. TRUE statements about "pulled elbow" or radial head subluxation include which of the following statements?

A. Radial head subluxation occurs when the radial head slips out from the lateral collateral ligament.

B. Most patients will have a palpable effusion and some ecchymosis at the site.

C. Classically, the child will hold the elbow in slightly flexed position with the hand pronated.

D. Radiographs should be ordered when this injury is suspected.

E. The flexion and supination method has been proven to be the superior method.

#58
Answer: C

Radial head subluxation is a common pediatric injury. Median age of presentation is 2 years of age. It's caused by forceful longitudinal traction on the radius, which displaces the radial head underneath the annular ligament, causing the ligament to become entrapped in the radiocapitellar joint.

Prior to attempting reduction, the provider should ensure that the history and physical exam are consistent with the diagnosis. On exam, the patient usually refuses to move the arm and keeps it slightly flexed at the elbow with hand pronation. There may be some tenderness; however, obvious deformity, bruising, or effusion should not be present. Radiographs are almost always normal and should not routinely be obtained.

Hyperpronation or supination and flexion of the arm will reduce the injury. Some studies have demonstrated the hyperpronation technique to be less painful and more effective. A successful reduction will result in the child moving the arm normally, generally with resolution of the pain within half an hour of the reduction. If diagnosis is unclear or reduction unsuccessful after 3-4 attempts, obtain a radiograph to rule out fracture, immobilize the arm with elbow at 90 degree flexion, and arrange orthopedic follow up.

- Aylor M et al. Reduction of pulled elbow. NEJM 2014; 371:e32.

#59

You prepare to examine a patient with complaints of right shoulder pain. TRUE statements about shoulder anatomy and shoulder complex injuries include which of the following?

A. The shoulder complex is composed of 2 bones and 2 joints.

B. The anteriorposterior (AP) and lateral view fulfill the American College of Radiology's standard for plain radiographs of the shoulder.

C. A posterior sternoclavicular dislocation is excluded by a normal plain radiograph.

D. Of plain x-ray views, the axillary view is most helpful in diagnosing posterior shoulder dislocations.

E. Both Bankart and Hill-Sachs lesions are equally visible on plain radiographs.

#59
Answer: D

The shoulder is comprised of three bones (clavicle, humerus, and scapula) and three joints (sternoclavicular, acromioclavicular, and glenohumeral). The American College of Radiology recommends obtaining three views: the AP view, axillary view, and the scapular Y view. A posterior sternoclavicular dislocation is very uncommon, but when present, can cause mediastinal damage resulting in airway and neurovascular compromise. If it is suspected, then a CT scan must be performed as plain films are not sufficiently sensitive in ruling out the diagnosis. Clavicle fractures that are open, occur in high-functioning athletes, produce significant skin-tenting, are intra-articular, or result in > 20mm of shortening may require operative intervention.

While anterior shoulder dislocations can frequently be diagnosed clinically, posterior shoulder dislocations are much more difficult to diagnose and are frequently missed on AP view. Axillary view is the most helpful in making the diagnosis. Bankart and Hill-Sachs lesions are common bony injuries that occur with anterior shoulder dislocations. Bankart lesions may cause a fracture of the glenoid rim, but it typically just results in damage to the cartilage and soft tissue structures, such as the labrum and anterior capsule, which are only visualized on MRI. Hill-Sachs lesions are the result of a compression fracture of the posterior aspect of the humeral head.

. Pescatore R, et al. Managing shoulder injuries in the emergency department: fracture, dislocation, and overuse. Emergency Medicine Practice 2018; 20, 6.

#60

Your patient has multiple lacerations on the palm and digits of his non-dominant hand which will benefit from a regional block prior to repair. TRUE statements about digital and wrist blocks include which of the following?

A. A potential advantage of the dorsal, traditional approach to the digital block (rather than the volar approach) is that there is only a single injection.

B. To block the radial nerve, the scaphoid and the ulnar styloid must be identified as anatomic landmarks.

C. To block the median nerve, identify the palmaris longus, and inject between this tendon and the flexor carpi ulnaris.

D. To block the ulnar nerve, first identify the ulnar styloid and the flexor carpi ulnaris tendon.

E. To reverse the cardiotoxic effects of a local anesthetic that has been inadvertently injected intravascularly, administer n-acetylcysteine.

#60
Answer: D

Peripheral nerve blocks reduce the risk of anesthetic toxicity and cause less tissue distortion. A digital nerve block, approached either via a dorsal or volar technique, can be helpful for patients with superficial lacerations to a single finger. The dorsal approach involves two injections on either side of the finger whereas the volar approach involves just one.

The landmarks that need to be identified for a radial nerve block include the radial artery and radial styloid. The needle is inserted radial to the radial artery at the level of the radial styloid and again subcutaneously along the dorsum of the wrist. The landmarks for the median nerve block include the palmaris longus and flexor carpi radialis. The needle is inserted 2.5 cm proximal to the wrist crease between these two tendons. To block the ulnar nerve, the needle is inserted under the flexor carpi ulnaris tendon, just above the ulnar styloid, and again subcutaneously along the dorsal aspect of the wrist, distal to the ulnar styloid.

Local anesthetic toxicity causes neurotoxicity and cardiotoxicity, which can result in seizure and cardiovascular collapse. Toxicity typically occurs due to accidental intravascular administration. This can be prevented by using local anesthetic formulations with epinephrine, which decreases systemic absorption and produces early symptoms if injected intravascularly. Treatment includes IV administration of 20% lipid emulsion.

• https://www.nejm.org/doi/full/10.1056/NEJMvcm1400191 (video link) Chandrasoma J et al. Peripheral nerve blocks for hand procedures. NEJM 2018;:379 e15

PEDIATRICS

#61

In room 3, there is a 3 year old male who placed a bean up his nose, and in room 4, there is a 4 year old who complains of ear pain after he believes an insect crawled into the canal. TRUE statements about foreign bodies in the nose and ear include which of the following statements?

A. The majority of retained foreign bodies in the ear and nose must be emergently removed.

B. Since the object in the nose is a bean, your first choice in technique for removal should be irrigation.

C. Irrigation as a method of removal would also be contraindicated if it is a magnet or battery.

D. A complication that may occur after foreign body removal from the ear is sinusitis.

E. The likelihood of success for retrieval of the foreign body in an outpatient setting increases with each additional attempt, up to three tries.

#61
Answer: C

Ear canal and nasal foreign bodies are commonly placed by children or adults with mental disabilities. Though certain objects, such as magnets and batteries, can cause serious tissue damage within hours and should be removed emergently, most foreign bodies do not require emergent removal.

Irrigation is a useful technique for removal in most situations (although rarely for nasal foreign bodies); however, it should be avoided with hygroscopic foreign bodies, such as beans, that will swell with water exposure, battery or magnet foreign bodies that cause more tissue damage when wet, and tympanic membrane perforations. Though a variety of methods and instruments can be utilized for foreign body removal, a few scenarios can be more easily managed with some specific recommendations: drowning an insect prior to its removal from an ear canal, using a combination of a topical decongestant (0.05% oxymetazoline) and an anesthetic agent (4% lidocaine) a few minutes prior to nasal foreign body removal, and removal of impacted ear canal foreign bodies under general anesthesia to minimize the severe pain and complications associated with the procedure.

Retained foreign bodies in the external auditory canal can cause complications, such as hearing loss, infection, and ear pain, whereas retained nasal foreign bodies can lead to sinusitis. The most common complications of foreign object removal are local tissue trauma. The success of foreign body removal depends not only upon the shape, size, and texture of the object, but the presence or absence of infection, duration the object has been in place, and the patient's anatomy. Also, the likelihood of foreign object removal decreases with each attempt in the outpatient setting.

- Friedman EM. Removal of foreign bodies from the ear and

nose. NEJM 2016; 374: e7.

#62

You are in the pediatric ED and are seeing a 15 year old girl with acne vulgaris that has not responded initial therapies, such as salicylic acid and benzoyl peroxide. She has many inflammatory lesions over her face, chest and back. Which of the following statements about the diagnosis and management of acne vulgaris is TRUE?

A. She should avoid caffeine and greasy foods, because these are causative in the pathogenesis of acne.

B. Acne should not persist into adulthood, and thus, if it does, a malignancy evaluation should be performed.

C. Polycystic ovarian disease (PCOS) is a risk factor for acne.

D. Patients should be counseled to scrub their face with an astringent several times a day.

E. There is no role for systemic antibiotics in managing severe acne.

#62
Answer: C

Acne is an inflammatory disorder of the pilosebaceous unit that predominantly affects teenagers, though it can often persist into adulthood. It's caused by a combination of inflammation, hyperkeratinization of hair follicles, and increased sebum production. Risk factors include a positive family history, metabolic syndrome, PCOS, and certain medication use (e.g., steroids, progestin-only contraceptives, lithium). Patients with severe/refractory symptoms, especially if abrupt onset, or females with signs of androgen excess should receive a hormonal work-up to evaluate for conditions such as PCOS or gonadal tumors.

No dietary recommendations can be made at this time, though patients should be taught to follow a skin care routine (e.g., limiting washing to twice a day, using gentle skin cleansers, avoiding astringents and scrubs). Treatment is guided by the severity of presentation. Combination therapy with a benzoyl peroxide-containing antimicrobial agent and a topical retinoid is recommended as initial management of mild-to-severe inflammatory acne. Cases that do not respond to topical therapies may improve the addition of oral antibiotics for 3 to 4 months or combined oral contraceptives and spironolactone, if female. Isotretinoin can be considered for patients with refractory or severe nodulocystic acne; however, the FDA mandates adherence to a strict monitoring program while using this medication because of its highly teratogenic side effects.

- Zaenglein AL. Acne vulgaris. NEJM 2018; 379: 1343-52.

#63

You are caring for a 15 year old female whose initial complaint was abdominal pain but now complains of contractions while waiting in the pediatric ED. TRUE statements about the management of an unexpected delivery in the ED include which of the following?

A. Nearly 1/3 of infants require special assistance at birth from medical providers during delivery.

B. If the neonate's heart rate is less than 130bpm, then bag-valve-mask should be initiated.

C. If bag-valve-mask and positive pressure ventilation are going to be initiated, the pulse oximetry monitoring should be placed on the neonate's left arm to obtain post-ductal saturations.

D. The two thumb technique for chest compressions at 3:1 is now the preferred compression method in a newborn.

E. The American Heart Association now recommends routine tracheal intubation in the setting of a depressed newborn with meconium-stained amniotic fluids.

#63
Answer: D

90% of infants do not require any assistance to successfully transition from intrauterine to extrauterine life at birth and only 1% need extensive resuscitation. At first evaluation (1 minute of life), assess the ABCs of the neonate including appearance, breathing, and color/cry. Bag-valve-mask should be initiated if the neonate's heart rate is less than 100 beats per minute or the respiratory rate is greater than 40-60 breaths per minute. The pulse oximetry probe should be placed on the right upper extremity to obtain preductal saturations. The two-thumb technique, where thumbs are placed on lower third of sternum and fingers on the infant's back, should be initiated if the heart rate is less than 60 beats per minute and the neonate is unresponsive to ventilatory support. The American Heart Association no longer recommends routine tracheal intubation in the setting of a depressed newborn with meconium-stained amniotic fluids.

• LLSA 2019 article - Gupta AG, Adler MD. Management of an unexpected delivery in the ED. Vol 17; 2; 89-98.

#64
A 17 year old female who denies any possibility of pregnancy presents with abdominal pain that is colicky and occurs every 3 minutes. During your exam, you note that a fetus is crowning and she is in active labor. TRUE statements about the management of an unexpected delivery in the ED include which of the following?

A. A standardized checklist of supplies and equipment necessary for a precipitous delivery is helpful as the event is rare in occurrence

B. If the baby has poor tone and is premature, the baby may stay with the mother.

C. Most neonatal cardiac arrest is due to hypovolemia.

D. Delayed cord clamping is no longer recommended.

E. Epinephrine should be administered if the heart rate is below 100 bpm

#64
Answer: A

Precipitous delivery in the emergency department is a rare occurrence and a standardized checklist of supplies and equipment is helpful. Important historical questions to ask include: whether the mother had prenatal care, gestational age, number of babies expected, and any pregnancy-related complications. These questions may help the provider assemble the appropriate personal necessary for the delivery. If possible, separate teams to manage the mother and newborn should be present. Upon delivery, if the neonate: (1) is term gestation, (2) has good tone, and (3) is breathing or crying, the newborn many stay with mother. In all other cases, the neonate should be taken to a pre-heated radiant warmer for further evaluation. Delayed cord clamping is now recommended for preterm and term infants who do not need resuscitation as it is associated with decreased need for postnatal transfusion, a lower incidence of necrotizing enterocolitis, and less intraventricular hemorrhage.

If resuscitation is necessary, the focus during the first minute of life should be on initiating ventilation as neonatal cardiac arrest is typically due to asphyxia. Volume expansion and epinephrine are administered if heart rate remains below 60 bpm despite intubation and chest compressions. It can be given at a dose of 0.01 – 0.03 mg/kg IV or 0.05 – 0.1 mg/kg via endotracheal tube.

. LLSA 2019 - Gupta AG, Adler MD. Management of an unexpected delivery in the emergency department. 2016; 17: 2:89-98.

#65

A 16 year old female delivers a pre-term infant with poor tone and cry in your emergency department. TRUE statements about the management of the newborn with respiratory compromise include which of the following?

A. A pulse oximetry probe should be placed on the left lower extremity because this would be preductal.

B. Resuscitation of all infants should be initiated with high oxygen concentrations.

C. A newborn may have a preductal saturation of 60-70% in the tenth minute of life, and this may be appropriate.

D. If the heart rate remains below 60 bpm after placement of an advanced airway, chest compressions at a ratio of 3 compressions: 1 breath for a synchronized rate of 120 events per minute should be initiated.

E. Heart rate is not a sensitive marker of effective ventilations during resuscitation.

#65
Answer: D

If a newborn has signs of respiratory compromise or airway obstruction, the airway should be adjusted by applying a chin lift or jaw thrust and/or airway secretions should be suctioned. If the neonate remains depressed, positive pressure ventilation via bag valve mask at a rate of 40-60 breaths per minute should be imitated. A pulse oximetry probe should be placed on the right upper extremity to obtain preductal saturations. Initially, low oxygen concentrations (FiO_2 21-30%) should be used and titrated up to achieve expected preductal saturations for corresponding minute of life. In the first minute of life, it is appropriate for newborns to have preductal oxygen saturations between 60-70%. They gradually increase to 85-95% by the tenth minute of life. A neonate's heart rate is one of the most sensitive markers of effective ventilations during resuscitation and it helps guide escalations in management. If the heart rate remains below 60 bpm after placement of an advanced airway, chest compressions at a ratio of 3 compressions: 1 breath for a synchronized rate of 120 events per minute should be initiated.

• LLSA 2019 - Gupta AG, Adler MD. Management of an unexpected delivery in the emergency department. 2016;17:2 89-98.

#66

In 2018, Kuppermann et al published a study in the New England Journal of Medicine that compared fluid types and rapid or slow rates of infusion in the management of pediatric diabetic ketoacidosis (DKA). Which of the following statements is TRUE?

A. Aggressive fluid resuscitation is associated with a greater degree of cerebral edema.

B. Aggressive fluid resuscitation decreases hospital lengths of stay.

C. Slow fluid resuscitation results in increased serious adverse events.

D. No significant differences were found among the treatment groups with respect to decline in Glasgow Coma Scale (GCS) or intelligence quotient (IQ) scores.

#66
Answer: D

It used to be believed that clinically apparent brain injury in pediatric DKA was due to rapid fluid resuscitation that resulted in decreased serum osmolality and brain swelling. However, more recent theories suggest that the brain edema is a secondary effect, rather than a cause, of the brain injury that develops due to the cerebral hypoperfusion, reperfusion and neuroinflammation that occur during the disease course and treatment. Kuppermann et al performed a randomized controlled, multicenter trial that sought to compare normal and half-normal saline in addition to rapid and slow rates of their infusion in pediatric DKA patients. The primary outcome was the neurological status during the treatment. Secondary outcomes included short-term memory, clinically apparent brain injury, as well as memory and IQ after recovery of DKA. Only 3.5% of patients had a decline in GCS, and only 0.9% had clinically apparent brain injury. There were no clinically significant differences among the treatment groups for all measures including serious adverse events. Compared to half normal saline, the normal saline group had a higher incidence of hyperchloremic acidosis, hypocalcemia, and hypophosphatemia.

- Kuppermann N et al. Clinical trial of fluid infusion rates for pediatric diabetic ketoacidosis. NEJM 2018; 378:2275-87.

#67

In 2017, the American Heart Association released a revised version of the 2004 guidelines for the diagnosis, treatment, and long-term management of Kawasaki Disease (KD). According to the guidelines, which of the following patients should be worked up for incomplete KD?

A. 10 year old girl with fever for 6 days and no other clinical criteria.

B. A 5 month old with fever for 7 days without any other clinical criteria and no other explanation for the fever.

C. A 2 year old with fever for 3 days and thrombocytopenia.

D. An 8 year old with fever, chest pain, and cough for 4 days.

E. All of the above

#67
Answer: B

Kawasaki Disease is classically diagnosed by the presence of 5 or more days of fever (typically greater than 39°C and remittent) in addition to at least 4 of the 5 principal clinical criteria which include: redness and swelling of the hands and feet with or without periungual desquamation, diffuse maculopapular rash, bilateral conjunctivitis without exudate, oral fissuring or erythema, and unilateral cervical lymphadenopathy (least common). The diagnosis can also be made with only 4 days of fever present, if the extremity changes are one of the four criteria present.

KD can be viewed as a disease spectrum and is clinically difficult to diagnose as all clinical features do not present at the same time or may not manifest at all. Incomplete KD should be considered in children with 5 days or more of fever as well as 2 or 3 compatible clinical criteria or infants under six months of age with 7 days or more of unexplained fevers. Due to the varying presentations, children with incomplete KD often have delayed diagnosis and substantial increased risks of developing coronary artery aneurysms. Diagnostic dilemmas often occur in infants less than 6 months of age with prolonged fever, and when rashes are mistakenly attributed to antibiotic reactions.

•   McCrindle BW et al. AHA Scientific Statement: Diagnosis, Treatment, and Long-term management of Kawasaki Disease. Circulation 2017; 1355:e929-999.

#68
A 15 year old male and a 5 year old male present to the ED separately with a chief complaint of a limp. TRUE statements about pediatric non-traumatic hip pathology include which of the following?

A. The patient with a hip effusion will often present with internal rotation.

B. Synovial fluid cell counts can reliably differentiate septic arthritis from Lyme arthritis.

C. The lack of a history of an erythema migrans rash precludes the diagnosis of Lyme arthritis.

D. Osteosarcomas are the most common pediatric primary bone cancer and Ewing sarcomas are the second most common.

E. Leukemia does not present with leg pain and limp.

#68
Answer: D

Pediatric non-traumatic hip pathology includes transient synovitis, Legg-Calve-Perthes disease (LCPD), slipped capital femoral epiphysis (SCFE), osteoarticular infections, and malignancy. Classically, patients with hip pathology including hip effusion, hemarthrosis, or hip fracture will keep their affected hip in flexion, abduction, and external rotation. Limitation to internal rotation is indicative of hip joint space disease.

Lyme arthritis is challenging to diagnose as many patients may lack the classic erythema migrans rash, and synovial fluid cell counts are not markedly different than those found in septic arthritis. Recommendations are to send serum Lyme serologies on patients diagnosed with septic arthritis in endemic areas or if other signs or symptoms of disseminated Lyme disease are present. Antibiotic treatment with amoxicillin for children under 8 years of age or doxycycline for older patients is the mainstay of management.

Malignancy is an infrequent cause of non-traumatic pediatric hip pathology and plain radiographs are the first line for evaluation. Classic findings for linear new bone growth help identify osteosarcoma and Ewing sarcomas, which are the first and second most common primary pediatric bone cancers respectively. Leukemia causes bone pain due to marrow expansion and typically presents with concurrent systemic symptoms such as lymphadenopathy, bruising, and hepatosplenomegaly. Laboratory analysis is often unhelpful for diagnosis of sarcomas but will be abnormal when bone marrow suppression or peripheral blasts are present in leukemia.

• LLSA 2019 article - Wagner Neville DN, Zuckerbraun N. Pediatric nontraumatic hip pathology. Vol. 17, 1: 13-28.

#69

A 7 year old male is brought in by his mother for a limp. Your differential diagnosis is broad and you are considering the use of plain radiographs, ultrasound, and MRI to clinch the diagnosis and etiology of the limp. TRUE statements of the limping child include which of the following?

A. The main use of hip sonography in non-traumatic hip pathology is to differentiate between a sterile and pyogenic effusion.

B. Comparison views are of no help when obtaining plain radiographs of the hip.

C. The usual age range of patients who present with slipped capital femoral epiphysis (SCFE) is 4 - 9.

D. Klein's line can help you diagnose osteosarcoma.

E. Patients with SCFE and underlying endocrinopathy are at increased risk for bilateral slips.

#69
Answer: E

It is important to obtain comparison anterior-posterior and frog-leg views of the full pelvis and bilateral hips when obtaining plain radiographs. The main use of hip sonography is for detection of an effusion as it is superior to radiographs. Sonography cannot differentiate between sterile and pyogenic effusions. An anterior-posterior fluid collection in the joint capsule that is greater than 5mm, or 2mm larger when compared to the contralateral hip, is diagnostic of a joint effusion.

Slipped capital femoral epiphysis (SCFE) is characterized by the slippage of the femoral head from the femoral neck through the physeal plate. The condition has a male predominance, typically presents between the ages of 10 – 16y, and is most commonly due to mechanical overload from obesity. There should be a concern for an underlying endocrinopathy, such as hypothyroidism or growth hormone deficiency, when it presents outside of the typical age range. Bilateral SCFE are more frequent in patients with underlying endocrinopathies. The typical onset is subacute and many patients present with pain referred to the knee or a limp. The diagnosis can be made on plain radiographs by drawing "Klein's line" along the superior aspect of the femoral neck in the AP view. If the line does not intersect the epiphysis of the femoral head then SCFE is present. This is only 60% sensitive; however, the sensitivity of the test can be significantly improved by measuring more than a 2mm difference in the additional epiphyseal width that lies lateral to Klein's line between hips. Patients should be made non-weight bearing and given immediate orthopedic consultation. Operative fixation is performed to prevent osteonecrosis of the femoral head.

• LLSA 2019 - Wagner Neville DN, Zuckerbraun N. Pediatric nontraumatic hip pathology.2016;17:13-28.

#70

A 4 year old male is being referred to your hospital for management of Legg-Calve-Perthes Disease (LCPD). The child appears well but is walking with a limp. TRUE statements regarding this disease entity include which of the following?

A. LCPD is thought to be due to bacterial translocation into the femoral head.

B. Blood supply to the femoral head is restored to normal within 1 to 2 years.

C. The disease process is more common in girls.

D. Approximately 50% of cases have bilateral involvement.

E. Treatment usually involves increased physical activity to promote weight loss.

#70
Answer: B

Legg-Calve-Perthes Disease (LCPD) is a self-limited, noninflammatory, aseptic idiopathic avascular necrosis of the proximal femoral epiphysis that occurs in children aged 2 – 12. It results in devascularization of the blood supply to the femoral head that returns to normal in 1 – 2 years. It has a male predominance and 10-15% have bilateral involvement. It has a subacute presentation and is not always painful. Though radiographs are diagnostic, they can be negative early, so MRI should be used to identify early disease. Radiographs will show the characteristic femoral head evolution from spherical to elliptical and irregular to fragmented. It results in degenerative joint changes and arthritis as an adult. Outpatient orthopedic referral should be provided and the goal of therapy is to prevent secondary degenerative changes. Management will range from decreased physical activity to surgical intervention.

- LLSA 2019 - Wagner Neville DN, Zucerbraun N. Pediatric nontraumatic hip pathology. 2017; 17:13-28.

#71

A 7 year old male presents with a fever and a limp. Last week, you saw him in the pediatric emergency department when his mother brought him in for cough and cold symptoms. While he liked you last week, today, he will not let you touch his leg and he cries whenever you make a movement towards him. You are concerned about septic arthritis, but you also consider osteomyelitis and transient synovitis. TRUE statements about non-traumatic pediatric hip pathologies include which of the following?

A. Joint fluid cultures in septic arthritis are positive in > 90%.

B. Laboratory finding in patients with osteomyelitis will be more similar to transient synovitis than septic arthritis.

C. If the synovial white blood count is less than 30,000 cells/µL, then septic arthritis is excluded.

D. MRI can help differentiate septic arthritis from osteomyelitis.

E. The Kocher criteria is used to differentiate septic arthritis from osteomyelitis.

#71
Answer: D

Transient synovitis is a diagnosis of exclusion and the most common diagnosis in pediatric patients with non-traumatic hip complaints. It is characterized by a self-limiting joint effusion that is caused by an unknown etiology and has no serious sequelae. It typically presents unilaterally and between the ages of 3 – 8 with an acute onset of pain. A history of a recent infection or minor trauma may be present and the child will be well-appearing and afebrile or with a low-grade temperature. The diagnosis is clinical, and resolution of symptoms with the ability to bear weight after treatment with an NSAID is reassuring. Management consists of close follow up, scheduled NSAID therapy, and return precautions for symptoms concerning for septic arthritis.

Osteoarticular infections can occur at any age though and most commonly occur from hematogenous spread. Septic arthritis and osteomyelitis may occur in isolation or concurrently. Patients with septic arthritis typically have a high fever and are toxic appearing. Diagnosis is made by isolation of a pathogen from the site of infection or from the blood if imaging shows evidence of inflammation at the site. Synovial fluid cultures are positive in less than 50% of septic arthritis cases. PCR use can increase their yield. In contrast to the low yield of blood and synovial fluid cultures in septic arthritis, bone cultures in osteomyelitis are positive in over 90% of cases. The Kocher criteria (refusal to bear weight, fever, ESR > 40mm/h, and serum WBC > 12,000 cells/μL) have classically been used to differentiate transient synovitis from septic arthritis. Patients with three or more criteria have over a 93% probability of septic arthritis. Recent analyses have shown that it is difficult to differentiate etiologies for hip effusions based on cell counts alone as the traditional cut off of synovial counts above 50,000 cells/μL have proven to be neither sensitive or specific for septic arthritis. MRI can help differentiate osteomyelitis from septic arthritis.

- LLSA 2019 - Wagner Neville DN, Zucerbraun N. Pediatric nontraumatic hip pathology. 2017; 17:13-28.

#72

You are in the pediatric emergency department and there is a 45 day old ex 35-week premature infant who is presenting with cyanosis and irregular breathing with increased tone that lasted 30 seconds in duration. This was the only episode. The episode was self-resolving and the child is now back to baseline. There was no cardiopulmonary resuscitation required. The physical examination in the ED is normal. You want to make the diagnosis of a brief resolved unexplained event (BRUE). However, this is NOT a BRUE because of which of the following?

A. The infant is not greater than 60 days of age.

B. There was only one event, and BRUE requires two occurrences.

C. The episode lasted greater than 15 seconds.

D. There was no CPR required.

E. The child appears well on physical examination.

#72
Answer: A

BRUE is a term used to describe an event in a patient greater than 60 days of age and less than 1 year where they are observed to have a sudden, brief, and now resolved episode of one or more of the following without an alternate explanation:

1. Cyanosis or pallor

2. Absent, decreased, or irregular breathing

3. Marked change in tone (hypertonia or hypotonia)

4. Altered level of responsiveness

The recommendations identify and provide evaluation and management guidelines for lower-risk patients who are identified by the following parameters:

1. Age > 60 days

2. Gestation age ≥ 32 weeks and postconceptional age ≥ 45 weeks

3. Occurrence of only 1 event (no prior events or recurrent events)

4. Duration < 60 seconds

5. No cardiopulmonary resuscitation by trained providers required

6. No concerning historical or physical examination findings

. LLSA 2019 reading list. Tieder JS et al. Brief resolved unexplained events (formerly apparent life-threatening events) and evaluation of lower risk infants: executive summary. Pediatrics 2016; 137.

#73

A 2 month old boy is brought to your emergency department after his mother noted pallor, increased tone and decreased responsiveness. You consider BRUE as the diagnosis. Which of the following management recommendations regarding lower risk BRUE is TRUE?

A. There is no role for shared decision-making to guide work-up and disposition for lower risk BRUE patients

B. Lower risk BRUE patients should have blood cultures drawn prior to discharge.

C. Lower risk BRUE patients should be discharged home with home cardio-respiratory monitors

D. Management recommendations for lower risk BRUE patients include that the provider may obtain a 12-lead ECG.

E. As the most common cause of a BRUE is gastroesophageal reflux, lower risk BRUE patients should be discharged with empiric acid suppression therapy

#73
Answer: D

Infants with BRUE should be well appearing, without abnormal vital signs, and without an alternate etiology for the event on history or physical (including gastroesophageal reflux or feeding difficulties). According to the management recommendations, lower risk BRUE patients should not receive "routine" labs, blood cultures, or an inborn error of metabolism work-up. Additionally, they should not be discharged on a home cardiorespiratory monitor or on anti-epileptic or acid suppression therapies. The authors do recommend educating the parents about BRUE and engaging in shared decision-making to help guide workup and disposition. A 12-lead ECG, pertussis testing, monitoring with pulse oximetry, and serial evaluations may be obtained by the provider.

. LLSA 2019 - Tieder JS, et al. Brief resolved unexplained events (formerly Apparent Life Threatening Events) and Evaluation of lower-risk infants: executive summary. Pediatrics 2016; 137.

PSYCHIATRY

#74

A 35 year old male is brought in by paramedics after a gunshot wound to the head that is reportedly self-inflicted. TRUE statements about gunshot wounds and suicide include which of the following?

A. A bullet fired from under the chin is suggestive of a suicide attempt. If the neck is hyperextended, the resulting injury is often nonlethal and spares the brain.

B. Suicide rates are steadily decreasing in the United States.

C. The vast majority of patients who commit suicide have a history of mental illness.

D. People who attempt suicide by firearms have a fatality rate of approximately 10%.

E. Most physicians ask patients about access to firearms when a patient expresses suicidal ideation.

#74
Answer: A

A bullet fired from under the chin is suggestive of a suicide attempt. If the neck is hyperextended, the resulting injury is often nonlethal and spares the brain. Suicide rates have substantially increased across the United States in all age groups between 10 and 75 years of age over the past two decades. Most people who die by suicide today have no known history of mental illness. It is thought that suicide is more of an impulsive act rather than a well-deliberated decision. Elements that increase impulsivity, such as substance abuse, may contribute to the action.

Most physicians do not ask patients about firearm access, even if suicidal ideation is expressed. As the fatality rate of attempted suicide by firearm is 85% compared to the 2% by poisoning or overdose, reducing access to guns during a period of crisis can be a potentially lifesaving intervention. This can be achieved by counseling patients or their families about safe firearm storage or voluntary firearm removal from the home. Additionally, 13 states provide legal avenues, under Extreme Risk Protection Orders (aka Red Flag laws), through which access to firearms can be temporarily restricted.

- Sacks CA, et al. Case 31-2018: A 37 year old man with a self-inflicted gunshot wound. NEJM 2018; 379:1464-72.

#75

A 50 year old homeless, alcoholic male is brought in by paramedics for public intoxication and suicidal ideation. Which of the following statements about the management of suicidal patients in the ED is TRUE?

A. Even though the patient is intoxicated, the patient may be assessed for suicidal risk.

B. Less than 1% of all adult ED patients, regardless of chief complaint, have had recent suicidal ideation or behaviors.

C. The Joint Commission requires suicide screening and assessment for patients with primary emotional or behavioral disorders as presenting symptoms.

D. Prior to obtaining collateral information from relevant sources, obtaining consent from the patient is mandatory.

E. "Contracting for safety" prevents suicide and is recommended.

#75
Answer: C

This paper's guidelines only apply to adult patients who are clinically sober and have capacity. Regardless of chief compliant, approximately 10% of all adult ED patients have had recent suicidal ideation or behaviors. Patients with presenting symptoms of emotional or behavioral disorders are required to have suicide screening and assessment by the Joint Commission. Though "contracting for safety" is not recommended as it has not been shown to prevent suicide, "safety planning," which involves creating a personalized plan to help the patient cope and seek help during a time of crisis, is encouraged. This involves identifying warning signs, accessible follow-up, and emergency contacts. All patients should be provided the phone number to the National Suicide Prevention Hotline (1-800-273-TALK [8255]).Management of the intoxicated, suicidal patient can be difficult in the ED. Key points include:

- Obtaining appropriate collateral resources is particularly important. Although asking for permission to contact relevant sources enhances rapport, consent is not required (to protect the individual (or public) from a serious and imminent safety threat).

- Routine diagnostic testing including laboratory or radiographic studies has not been shown to be beneficial.

- Alcohol use raises risk of suicide with more serious thoughts, plans, and attempts.

. LLSA 2018 article - Betz ME, Boudreaux ED. Managing suicidal patients in the ED. Ann Emerg Med 2016;67:276-282.

#76

You are seeing a 25 year old female with persecutory delusions and auditory hallucinations. TRUE statements about psychotic disorders include which of the following?

A. This age group (20-30) is atypical for the onset of idiopathic psychotic disorders, such as schizophrenia, bipolar, and schizoaffective disorders.

B. Features that suggest a secondary psychosis, rather than the idiopathic psychotic disorders, include a gradual onset of illness without a clear precipitant.

C. Neurotransmitters implicated in the psychotic disorders include serotonin.

D. Immune encephalitis, secondary to antibodies against the NR1 subunit of the NMDA glutamate receptor (which can cause symptoms similar to schizophrenia) are associated with ovarian teratomas.

E. The diagnosis of psychotic disorders hinges upon serologic assays.

#76
Answer: D

Psychiatric disorders including bipolar disorder, schizophrenia, and depression with psychotic symptoms, most commonly begin in the age group of 20-30. In contrast, delusional disorders usually occur in middle age, and psychosis secondary to Alzheimer's begins during senescence. Secondary psychosis has several distinguishing features compared to idiopathic type which include: an abrupt onset of symptoms without clear precipitants, a rapid decline in functional status, a lack of family history of psychotic disorders, and a history of headaches, seizures, or hallucinations. The main neurotransmitters implicated in the pathophysiology of psychotic disorders are dopamine, glutamate, and GABA. Immune encephalitidies produce psychotic symptoms similar to those in schizophrenia. Encephalitis due to antibodies against the NR1 subunit of the NMDA glutamate receptor most commonly occurs with ovarian teratomas. Despite the mechanism of psychotic disorders, the diagnosis is predominantly clinical and neuroimaging, EEG, genotyping, toxicologic, and serological assays are supportive. Early diagnosis is paramount, as early detection and treatment of schizophrenia improves overall prognosis with decreased burden of this chronic disease.

• Lieberman JA, First MB. Psychotic Disorders, NEJM 2018:379:270-80.

PULMONARY

#77

A 55 year old male with history of colon cancer post-operative day #8 from his total colectomy presents in cardiac arrest. You suspect a pulmonary embolism (PE). TRUE statements about PE include which of the following?

A. PE has been categorized into either non-massive versus massive PE.

B. Massive PE is defined by RV strain without signs of hemodynamic instability.

C. For the patient in cardiac arrest and evidence of PE, thrombolytics are indicated.

D. The studies on submassive PE have collectively used standardized definitions and a universally accepted protocol.

E. Thrombolytic use for submassive PE has literature to support no increased risk of bleeding.

#77
Answer: C

Acute PE is categorized as nonmassive, submassive, and massive. Nonmassive PE has no evidence of right ventricular strain (defined by echocardiographic signs or laboratory biomarkers), and no hemodynamic instability. Submassive PE has evidence of right ventricular strain but no hemodynamic instability. Occlusive thromboemboli that produce hemodynamic instability are categorized as massive PE.

Treatment involves anticoagulation and thrombolysis. Massive PE is an indication for using thrombolysis with one meta-analysis showing decreased risk of death and recurrent PE. However, the evidence for using thrombolysis in submassive PE is inconsistent due to the heterogeneity in the literature in how the condition is defined, selected primary outcomes, and treatment protocols. The risks, such as major bleeding (much more likely in the elderly), and benefits, such as decreased long-term risk for pulmonary hypertension, must be weighed appropriately. Contraindications to thrombolytics include suspected dissection, ischemic stroke within the past 3 months, known structural cerebrovascular disease, and prior intracranial hemorrhage. There is some evidence that outcomes can be improved with half-dose thrombolytics and catheter directed treatments, but further studies are needed.

- LLSA 2019 article - Long B, Koyfman A. Current controversies in thrombolytic use in acute pulmonary embolism. JEM 2016; 51:37-44

#78

A 78 year old female who carries a diagnosis of idiopathic pulmonary fibrosis (IPF) presents with increasing dyspnea on exertion and increasing home oxygen requirements. TRUE statements about IPF and its diagnosis and management include which of the following statements?

A. IPF is generally a disease of the young.

B. There are no treatments that have been found to decrease the progression of illness.

C. Prednisone should not be used for treatment.

D. Pulmonary function testing usually demonstrates a high functional vital capacity (FVC).

E. Patients with IPF will usually complain of a chronic purulent cough.

#78
Answer: C

IPF is the most common type of idiopathic interstitial pneumonia that is defined by a chronic, progressive, fibrotic interstitial lung disease that is not secondary to infection or cancer. Interstitial lung disease describes a family of diseases with a combination of cellular proliferation, interstitial inflammation, and fibrosis that occur within the alveolar wall. IPF primarily occur in older adults and is often misdiagnosed and mismanaged. New treatments, including medications such as nintedanib and pirfenidone have been shown to be safe and effective for slowing the progression of illness. Other immunosuppressive therapies, such as prednisone in combination with azathioprine and oral N-acetylcysteine, have been shown to increase mortality by a factor of 9 and should not be used for treatment.

Clinically, IPF presents with external dyspnea, non-purulent cough, and general fatigue. Physical examination demonstrates bilateral "Velcro-like" crackles. Pulmonary function testing will show low diffusing capacity of the lung for carbon monoxide (DLCO) and normal or low FVC. Diagnosis is supported through high-resolution CT, although surgical biopsy is the gold standard. Supplemental home oxygen is strongly recommended due to improved external dyspnea and improved exercise tolerance.

- Lederer DJ, Martinez FJ. Idiopathic pulmonary fibrosis. NEJM 2018; 378:1811-23.

#79

In the evaluation of patients with pleural disease (e.g. pleural effusion, pneumothorax, hemothorax), which of the following statements is TRUE?

A. Light's criteria more accurately classifies transudative effusions than exudative effusion.

B. A large bore chest tube (36 Fr) is recommended for parapneumonic effusions.

C. A transudative effusion associated with CHF, hepatic failure, and renal failure are not poor prognostic markers.

D. A spontaneous pneumothorax should be treated with a small-bore (14 French) chest tube.

E. Pleural fluid is largely produced and absorbed by the visceral pleura.

#79
Answer: D

Light's criteria correctly identifies nearly all exudative effusions; however, 25% of transudates are misclassified as exudates. This is especially true for CHF patients on diuretics. Currently, guidelines are moving away from using large bore chest tubes. Current guidelines recommend using small bore (14-French) chest tubes for parapneumonic effusions, empyema, and pneumothorax. Pneumothorax may initially be treated with simple needle aspiration, or with supplemental oxygen with observation. If these initial measures fail, a small bore chest tube is recommended. Spontaneous pneumothorax recurrence rates exceed 50%. Pleural fluid is produced and absorbed primarily by the parietal pleura. Transudative effusions are most commonly caused by congestive heart failure, cirrhosis, and renal failure, which have an associated 1-year mortality rates of 50%, 25%, and 46%, respectively.

- Feller-Kopman D, Light R. Pleural disease. NEJM 2018; 378:740-51.

#80

You are now seeing a patient who has a history of chronic obstructive pulmonary disease (COPD) and presents with increased shortness of breath, chest pain, and cough productive of purulent sputum. You suspect an acute exacerbation of COPD. TRUE statements about this entity include all of the following EXCEPT:

A. Arrhythmias associated with COPD include multifocal atrial tachycardia

B. Bacterial infections account for 50% of acute exacerbations of COPD

C. Guidelines recommend that the target oxygen saturation is > 92%.

D. Recommended steroid treatment is prednisone 40mg for 5 days.

E. If the patient is intubated, high inspiratory flow rates are recommended.

#80
Answer: C

Multiple arrhythmias are associated with COPD including: atrial fibrillation/flutter, non-sustained/sustained ventricular tachycardia, and multifocal atrial tachycardia. Multifocal atrial tachycardia is an irregular, narrow rhythm with at least 3 distinct P-wave morphologies. Other EKG findings of COPD include right atrial enlargement and right ventricular hypertrophy. Approximately 50% of COPD exacerbations are caused by bacterial infections, such as *Haemophilus influenza, Streptococcus pneumoniae, and Moraxella*. Guidelines recommend target **oxygen saturation of 88-92%**. Medication management includes 40 mg oral prednisone for 5 days and antibiotics for 5-7 days in the non-critically ill patients. Lung protective strategies are recommended for mechanically intubated patients including: tidal volumes of 6 cc/kg ideal body weight, a high inspiratory flow, and longer expiratory times per breath.

. Holden V et al. Diagnosis and management of acute exacerbation of chronic obstructive pulmonary disease. Emergency Medicine Practice, October 2017: volume 19, no. 10.

RENAL AND VASCULAR

#81

You are seeing a 34 year old non-pregnant female with pyelonephritis. TRUE statements regarding pyelonephritis include which of the following?

A. If the patient is tolerating orals, the patient could be treated with 5 days of levofloxacin (750 mg per day).

B. Imaging may be indicated if there is a new decrease of GFR to 40 ml/min or lower.

C. Up to 20% of patients with pyelonephritis do not have bladder symptoms.

D. Fosfomycin is not recommended for pyelonephritis.

E. All of the above

#81
Answer: E

There are no consensus diagnostic criteria for pyelonephritis due its wide variety of presentations. Up to 20% of patients lack bladder symptoms, some are afebrile, and others have septic shock. Urine culture is the primary confirmatory diagnostic test. Imaging is not routinely recommended unless patient's present with any of the following: sepsis or septic shock, urine pH $\geq$ 7.0, known or suspected urolithiasis, or a new decrease in GFR to 40 ml/min or lower.

Treatment with antibiotics usually targets E. Coli; however, a growing prevalence of resistance to fluoroquinolones and trimethoprim-sulfamethoxazole complicates treatment. Referral to local antibiograms is recommended. In general, administration of a long-acting parental antimicrobial agents should be considered if greater than 10% resistance exists for the oral therapy. Recommendation for oral therapy include: levofloxacin 750mg daily for 5 days, standard or high dose extended release ciprofloxacin for 7 days, trimethoprim – sulfamethoxazole for 14 days, and oral beta-lactams for 10 to 14 days. It should be noted that nitrofurantoin and oral fosfomycin only concentrate in the bladder and should not be used to treat pyelonephritis (can be used in simple cystitis if consistent with local antibiogram).

. LLSA 2019 article - Johnson JR, Russo TA. Acute pyelonephritis in adults. NEJM 2018; 378:48-59.

#82

A 65 year old male with diabetes, hypertension, hyperlipidemia presents with right great toe gangrene. He has a history of rest pain, and you diagnose him with chronic limb-threatening ischemia. TRUE statements about his condition include which of the following?

A. Patients with chronic limb threatening ischemia have a low risk of associated cardiovascular disease, such as MI and stroke.

B. The majority of chronic limb threatening ischemia is due to aorto-iliac disease.

C. Recommended medical therapies include a statin, aspirin and control of blood pressure and glucose.

D. Physical exam findings may include rubror with elevation of the extremity.

E. Randomized controlled trials have definitively demonstrated the superiority of endovascular treatment over open surgical bypass.

#82
Answer: C

Chronic limb-threatening ischemia is defined by having any one of the following: ischemic rest pain lasting 2 or more weeks, non-healing wounds, or gangrene that is due to proven arterial occlusive disease. Patients are at a high risk of associated cardiovascular disease (4-year risk of MI is 10% and 4-year risk of stroke is 8%), and death. The majority of chronic limb-threatening ischemia is due to infrainguinal arterial occlusive disease. The smoker and diabetic subgroups often have associated aortoiliac and infrapopliteal disease, respectively. On history, pain is worse with elevation and lessens with dependency. Physical examination is typically notable for: elevation pallor, dependent rubror, absent pulses, thin or shiny skin, hair loss, and increased capillary refill time.

Recommended medical therapies for chronic limb-threatening ischemia include a statin, aspirin, and control of blood pressure and glucose. These therapies, along with smoking cessation, have been shown to reduce limb-related outcomes and cardiovascular events. Diagnostic testing typically involves imaging such as, duplex ultrasound, CTA, or MRA to gain information about the location and extent of the disease. Treatment options for revascularization should only be used after infection, if present, has been treated. It includes both surgical and endovascular therapy with no clear superiority. Other causes of chronic limb threatening ischemia include: Buerger's disease, dissection, trauma, vasculitis, fibromuscular dysplasia, adventitial cystic disease, and physiological entrapment syndromes.

• Farber A. Chronic limb-threatening ischemia. NEJM 2018; 379:171-180.

#83

According to the 3SITES study that was conducted to compare different insertion sites for central venous catheters, which of the following statements is TRUE?

A. Subclavian vein catheterization was associated with the highest infection rate.

B. Subclavian vein catheterization was associated with the highest thrombotic rate.

C. Subclavian vein catheterization was associated with the highest pneumothorax rate.

D. The use of ultrasonographic guidance during catheter insertion was randomized.

E. The authors also compared the central catheters to peripherally inserted central catheters (PICC).

#83
Answer: C

The trial concluded that subclavian vein catheterization (SVC) was associated with a lower risk of bloodstream infection and symptomatic thrombosis. However, the SVC was found to have a higher risk of pneumothorax, compared to jugular and femoral vein catheterization. This was a well-done study with no patients lost to follow-up, similar baseline characteristics of all groups, adequate analysis methods, and standardized diagnostic testing for complications. There were several limitations to the study, including: lack of randomization of ultrasound use during catheter insertion, lack of chlorhexidine impregnated dressings or daily chlorhexidine bathing, and the study did not employ the use of peripherally inserted central venous catheters. When considering mechanical, infectious, and thrombotic complications equally, no particular insertion site was ideal.

• LLSA 2018 article - Parienti JJ et al. Intravascular complications of central venous catheterization by insertion site. NEJM 2015; 373:1220-9.

#84

You are seeing a 75 year old female with abdominal pain. The medical student who is shadowing you asks whether or not mesenteric ischemia is a possibility. With respect to mesenteric ischemia, which of the following statements is TRUE?

A. Arterial obstruction, the most common cause of mesenteric ischemia, has both acute and chronic forms.

B. Venous obstruction has both acute and chronic forms.

C. Dissection of the mesenteric vessel constitutes the vast majority of acute mesenteric ischemia.

D. Acute occlusion of at least two mesenteric vessels is necessary to cause mesenteric ischemia because of the rich collateral circulation that exists.

E. Serum biomarkers are diagnostic of acute mesenteric ischemia.

#84
Answer: A

Arterial obstruction is the most common cause of mesenteric ischemia and has both acute and chronic forms. Embolic occlusion accounts for about half of all cases of acute mesenteric ischemia (AMI), which is a surgical emergency. Another quarter to a third of cases is due to thrombotic occlusion of a previously stenosed mesenteric vessel, and dissection or inflammation of the artery account for < 5% of cases. A single vessel occlusion (typically the superior mesenteric artery) results in profound ischemia. The recommended diagnostic testing for AMI is CT angiography, as serum biomarkers are not reliable. Treatment options for AMI include thrombectomy, or angioplasty with stenting.

Almost all cases of chronic arterial mesenteric ischemia are caused by progressive atherosclerotic disease that affects the origins of the visceral vessel. These patients develop additional collateral networks over time and symptoms typically do not manifest until more than one primary vessel is occluded.

Mesenteric ischemia can also be caused by venous thrombosis in 5-15% of cases which results in impaired venous outflow, visceral edema, and abdominal pain. Venous obstruction is not categorized by acute or chronic forms, and almost all cases are related to thrombophilia, trauma, or local inflammatory changes of another organ system. The remaining cases of venous obstruction are related to cardiac insufficiency.

. LLSA 2019 article - Clair DG, Beach JM. Mesenteric ischemia. NEJM 2016; 374:959-68.

TOXICOLOGY

#85

A 30 year old patient presents with return of spontaneous circulation after cardiac arrest. The EKG in the ED demonstrates a wide complex tachycardia with a prolonged QTc interval, rightward shift of the QRS complex, and a positive R wave in lead aVR. There was an empty pill bottle of amitriptyline by her bedside. You suspect tricyclic antidepressant (TCA) overdose. TRUE statements about TCA overdose include which of the following?

A. The immunoassay to assess TCA ingestion provides a quantitative measure of the ingestion.

B. An R/S ratio in aVR > 0.6 and an R-wave height of > 3 mm is predictive of seizures and arrhythmias.

C. Sodium bicarbonate is indicated if the EKG demonstrates sinus tachycardia and a bundle branch block.

D. If a patient with a TCA overdose has refractory hypotension, the vasopressor of choice is dopamine.

E. Physostigmine is indicated if the QRS width exceeds 100ms.

#85
Answer: B

The immunoassay for TCA ingestion provides a qualitative measurement that is not specific for the number of drugs ingested or for a toxic ingestion. Additionally, multiple medications including diphenhydramine can cause false positive results. The clinically significant toxic dose for TCA is 10 to 20 mg/kg. There are several classic EKG findings of TCA overdose which include: sinus tachycardia, wide QRS complex prolonged QTc interval, prolonged PR interval, and rightward shifts of the QRS complex, especially the terminal portion as evidenced by a positive R wave in aVR. More specifically, a QRS width > 100ms is associated with seizures and > 160ms is associated with arrhythmias. In lead aVR, an R/S ratio > 0.6 and an R-wave height > 3mm are associated with both seizures and arrhythmias.

The mainstay of treatment is sodium bicarbonate which is indicated in patients with hemodynamic instability or a QRS width > 100ms. It provides sodium to stabilize myocardial sodium channels and alkalinizes the blood, which alter the cells' polarity, increases protein binding, which leads to reduced free drug levels. Norepinephrine or epinephrine are the preferred vasopressor agents in patients with refractory TCA hypotension, which is usually due to peripheral alpha-adrenergic blockade. Other treatment modalities include IV lipid emulsion, benzodiazepines for seizure, and several antiarrhythmics including: magnesium (in setting of prolonged QTc interval) and class IB agents (e.g. lidocaine). Hemodialysis or hemoperfusion are ineffective as TCAs are highly protein-bound resulting in a large volume of distribution. Class IA and IC agents should be avoided, class III agents (beta-blockers, amiodarone) can worsen hypotension, and physostigmine should only be reserved for pure anticholinergic toxidromes without QRS widening.

- Goldstein JN et al. Case 12-2018: A 30 year old woman with cardiac arrest.

Amy Kaji

NEJM 2018;378:1538-46.

#86

Your patient has sustained a snake bite to his hand. He believes that the snake was a rattlesnake. His hand appears to be edematous and there is circumferential swelling with redness associated with a bite mark. TRUE statements about snake envenomations include which of the following?

A. The only indigenous species of snakes in North America that are venomous are the Elapidae (coral snakes).

B. The predominant toxicity of pit viper venom is neurotoxic.

C. Copperhead bites are responsible for the highest mortality and morbidity rates in the US.

D. If you suspect compartment syndrome in the patient's hand, first-line treatment is fasciotomy.

E. The dosing of FabAV is the same, regardless of age (8-12 vials if cardiovascular collapse; otherwise 4-6 vials).

#86
Answer: E

The two major venomous North American indigenous snake subfamilies are Cortalineae (pit viper) and Elapidae (coral snake). The severity of snakebites depends on several factors ranging from the type of venom to the clothing worn by the patient. For example, pit viper venom is predominantly hemotoxic and can cause decreased fibrinogen and thrombocytopenia from fibrinolysis, increased platelet consumption, and rarely DIC.

Neurotoxicity is not associated with pit viper envenomations but varying neurologic symptoms, including fasciculations, weakness, and paresthesias have been reported. FabAV is indicated for pit viper envenomation with rapid progression of swelling or joint involvement, coagulopathy (increased PT, decreased fibrinogen, and thrombocytopenia), hemodynamic compromise, or late or recurrent coagulopathy. Dosing of FabAV is the same, regardless of age and is comprised of an initial bolus of 4-6 vials. 8-12 vials should be administered in the setting of cardiovascular collapse. After initial control has been achieved, maintenance dosing with antivenom is required, due to the long half-life of the venom. Antivenom, not fasciotomy, is the first-line treatment for compartment syndrome, as muscle necrosis caused by the envenomation will not be affected by removal of the surrounding fascia.

According to the US Poison Control, copperhead snakebites are the most commonly reported, but rattlesnake bites produce the highest mortality and morbidity rates. Coral snake venom is neurotoxic and binds muscarinic acetylcholine receptors at the neuromuscular junction. Though coral snake envenomations can cause a descending flaccid paralysis with bulbar symptoms such as diplopia or dysphagia, death is extremely rare. Tourniquet application and pressure immobilization are not recommended in the pre-hospital setting.

• Sheikh S, Leffers P. Emergency Department management of North American Snake Envenomations. September 2018; Vol 20, #9.

#87

A 29 year old female presents with nausea and vomiting. She is not pregnant and she is not diabetic. You suspect cannabis hyperemesis syndrome. TRUE statements about cannabinoids include which of the following?

A. The neuropsychiatric and addictive properties of cannabis are primarily due to the TRPV1 receptor.

B. There is no associated increased risk of stroke or TIA in regular users of cannabis.

C. There is no associated increased risk of myocardial infarction in regular users of cannabis.

D. Synthetic cannabinoids will not show up on routine urine drug screens.

E. Treatment of cannabis hyperemesis syndrome includes the administration of ice packs.

#87
Answer: D

The addictive and neuropsychiatric properties of cannabis are primarily due to delta-9-THC. The inhaled route has the shortest duration of action and effects can be seen within 3 minutes. Cannabis users who smoke at least once weekly have a higher risk of cerebrovascular events and a 5-fold increased risk of MI within the first hour of use. AKI and rhabdomyolysis have been noted with synthetic cannabinoid use, and cannabis intoxication is associated with metabolic abnormalities, such as hyperthermia, hyponatremia, hypokalemia, hypoglycemia, and metabolic acidosis. Synthetic cannabinoids have gained popularity because manufacturers are able to produce newer compounds that circumvent DEA designation as well as routine urine and serum drug screening tests. The mainstays for the treatment of cannabis hyperemesis syndrome are supportive therapies and cessation of cannabis use. Patients with cannabis hyperemesis syndrome are believed to crave hot showers because of activation of the TRPV1 receptor. Topical capsaicin applied to the torso may be used as an adjunctive therapy and works through a similar mechanism of action. Haloperidol at 2.5 mg IV can be considered for refractory vomiting associated with cannabis hyperemesis syndrome.

. Williams MV. Cannabinoids: emerging evidence in use and abuse. 2018; 20:8.

#88

You are caring for a patient who is frequently seen in the ED for alcohol intoxication. He appears to be intoxicated, but his alcohol level is undetectable and his head CT is unremarkable. You suspect a toxic alcohol ingestion with methanol, ethylene glycol, diethylene glycol, isopropanol, or propylene glycol. Which of the following is TRUE regarding toxic alcohols?

A. An increased serum osmolal gap must be present if the patient has a toxic alcohol ingestion.

B. An increased anion gap must be present if the patient has a toxic alcohol ingestion.

C. Coingested alcohol will accelerate the production of toxic metabolites and the onset of signs and symptoms.

D. Antidotal treatment with fomepizole is FDA approved for all of the toxic alcohols.

E. Alcohol dehydrogenase inhibitors should not be used for isopropanolol.

#88
Answer: E

Toxic alcohols include methanol, ethylene glycol, isopropanol, propylene glycol, and diethylene glycol. Except for isopropanol, the toxic alcohols are not directly toxic and their toxic effects result from their metabolites. Alcohol dehydrogenase performs the first oxidation of toxic alcohols into aldehydes (except for acetone, which is a ketone produced from isopropanol). These aldehydes are further oxidized by aldehyde dehydrogenase to form carboxylic acid metabolites: formic acid from methanol, oxalic and glycolic acid from ethylene glycol, 2-hydroxyethoxyacetic and glycolic acid from diethylene glycol, and lactic acid from propylene glycol.

Clinical symptoms vary greatly with the toxic alcohols but generally depress the sensorium and later produce organ dysfunction. Osmolal and anion gaps can help with diagnosis but cannot be used to definitely rule in or out a toxic alcohol ingestion. Classically, accumulation of the alcohol increases the osmolal gap, and later accumulation of organic acid anions increases the serum anion gap but this varies greatly depending on the course of intoxication.

Coingestion of ethanol delays production of toxic metabolites through competitive inhibition of alcohol dehydrogenase and can be used as an antidotal treatment, though it is not FDA approved for this indication. **Fomepizole (4-methylpyrazole), which inhibits alcohol dehydrogenase thereby decreasing toxic metabolite production, is an antidotal treatment that is FDA approved for ethylene glycol and methanol intoxication.** Fomepizole should not be used for isopropanol intoxication because it slows the removal of the toxic alcohol; supportive treatment is usually sufficient. Hemodialysis can remove toxic alcohols and their metabolites. This is an option for patients with severe metabolic acidosis, hemodynamic instability, vision problems (methanol ingestions), extremely high toxic alcohol levels, or acute kidney injury.

- Kraut JA, Mullins ME. Toxic alcohols. NEJM 2018; 378:270-80.

TRAUMA AND SURGERY

#89

You get a pre-hospital report about a 34 year old male who is being brought in by paramedics for a gun-shot wound to the chest and abdomen. He is hypotensive in the field. Which of the following statements about hemorrhagic shock is TRUE?

A. In the field, the patient should receive as many liters of saline as possible.

B. Hypotension is a very sensitive marker for hemorrhagic shock.

C. Ideally, blood product transfusion and resuscitation should be guided by measuring viscoelastic testing, such as thromboelastography or rotational thromboelastometry.

D. Blood products contain citrate, and massive transfusions can therefore lead to hypercalcemia.

E. Resuscitative Endovascular Balloon Occlusion of the Aorta (REBOA) has been shown definitively to decrease mortality in all trauma patients with hemorrhagic shock.

#89
Answer: C

Hemorrhagic shock causes high morbidity and mortality worldwide, with the majority caused by physical trauma. In the pre-hospital setting, it is important to limit fluid resuscitation as overzealous crystalloid resuscitation can dilute oxygen carrying capacity and clotting factor concentrations as well as worsen acidosis. Hypotension is a very insensitive marker for hemorrhagic shock as most patients have robust compensatory mechanisms until about 30% of the blood volume has been lost. Diagnostic testing of cellular hypoperfusion is performed by measuring base deficit and lactate from blood gas analysis. Additionally, viscoelastic testing such as thromboelastography or rotational thromboelastometry can be used to guide blood product resuscitation.

Massive transfusion protocols help assemble universal donor blood products along with calcium and tranexamic acid to the bedside. Transfusion of a 1:1:1 ratio of plasma, platelet and red cells appears to reduce short-term mortality. Blood products contain citrate, which can cause life-threatening hypocalcemia. Resuscitative Endovascular Balloon Occlusion of the Aorta (REBOA) may have a benefit in select patients with purely abdominal or pelvic bleeding but should not be used in all trauma patients with hemorrhagic shock.

. Cannon, JW. Hemorrhagic shock. NEJM 2018; 378:370-9.

#90

You are seeing several bleeding, hypotensive trauma patients simultaneously. TRUE statements about hemorrhage control include which of the following?

A. Part of damage control resuscitation involves achieving a normal blood pressure.

B. If a tourniquet is placed, it should be taken down with an assessment of the limb every two hours.

C. Due to trauma over-triage, Eastern Association for the Surgery of Trauma (EAST) recommends a higher threshold for trauma activation in the elderly.

D. When hemostatic agents such as Combat Gauze are used, there is no need for direct pressure, as long as the gauze is packed into the wound.

E. EAST does not recommend Tranexamic acid (TXA) in the trauma patient, because it has been associated with thromboembolic complications.

#90
Answer: B

Damage control resuscitation (DCR) is an approach to hemorrhage control that emphasizes achieving mechanical hemostasis, limiting crystalloid and artificial colloid administration, avoiding hypothermia, and allowing for permissive hypotension. The Eastern Association for the Surgery of Trauma (EAST) guidelines recommend a lower threshold for trauma activation and a higher level of care for geriatric trauma. A neurovascular exam should be performed prior to placement of a tourniquet. Time of tourniquet placement should be noted and takedown of the device should be performed every two hours for assessment. Hemostatic dressings such as Combat Gauze are considered first-line hemostatic agents. After they are packed into the wound, the provider should apply a minimum of 3-5 minutes of direct pressure and then apply a pressure dressing. Unstable pelvic fractures should have pelvic circumferential compression devices applied as a temporizing measure until definitive fixation is performed. EAST guidelines conditionally recommend the early use of TXA in the severely injured hemorrhaging patient.

• Boulger C, Yang B. Hemorrhage control: advances in trauma care. Trauma Reports 2018; 19:2.

#91

Your patient is being evaluated for blunt abdominal and head trauma. The patient is taking rivaroxaban for a prior unprovoked DVT. TRUE statements about this trauma patient include which of the following?

A. Application of the Canadian Head CT or New Orleans rule would be appropriate to determine whether the patient needs a head CT.

B. Eastern Association for the Surgery of Trauma (EAST) states that if a head CT is negative in an anticoagulated patient on warfarin, the patient can be discharged home.

C. The risk of delayed ICH in a person who is anti-coagulated is nearly 50%.

D. Concurrent alcohol intoxication has the potential to confound the thromboelastogram's (TEG's) utility.

E. FAST can definitively rule out solid organ injury.

#91
Answer: D

Clinical decision rules (e.g., Canadian CT Head rule, New Orleans criteria, Nexus-II criteria) do not apply to patients taking anticoagulation therapy, as this patient population was excluded during the derivation stage. EAST guidelines recommend patients anticoagulated with warfarin with supra-therapeutic INR and initial negative head CT to be admitted for observation, due to risk of delayed intracranial hemorrhage (DICH). Studies have shown a very low rate of DICH, making admission of all elderly anticoagulated patients not practical or economically feasible.

A thromboelastogram (TEG) provides an assessment of the coagulation cascade by measuring clot formation and viscoelasticity of whole blood under low shear stress. TEG had been shown to decrease mortality in patients requiring MTP; however, concurrent alcohol intoxication can potentially confound TEG's utility. The FAST exam may expedite operative intervention and improve mortality in a select group of patients; however, it cannot be used to definitively rule out solid organ, retroperitoneal, or bowel wall injury.

- Lawner BJ et al. Trauma mythology: looking beyond the ABCD and ATLS. Trauma Reports 2018; 19:no.5.

Made in the
USA
Columbia, SC